Oral Sciences

U0321457

Chief Editor

Zheng Sun

Contributors

Jingping Bai	Zhengxue Han	Xiaomei Hou
Xin Huang	Haiou Jia	Jingming Liu
Zhaochen Shan	Zheng Sun	Dongqing Wang
Rudong Xing	Xiaojiang Yang	

高等教育出版社·北京
HIGHER EDUCATION PRESS BEIJING

图书在版编目（CIP）数据

口腔科学 = Oral Sciences : 英文 / 孙正主编 .--

北京：高等教育出版社，2012.5
ISBN 978-7-04-034140-9

Ⅰ.①口… Ⅱ.①孙… Ⅲ.①口腔科学－医学院校－

教材－英文 Ⅳ.① R78

中国版本图书馆 CIP 数据核字（2012）第 034124 号

总　策　划　林金安　吴雪梅　席　雁

策划编辑　瞿德竑　　责任编辑　瞿德竑　　封面设计　张　楠　　责任印制　毛斯璐

出版发行	高等教育出版社	咨询电话	400 - 810 - 0598
社　　址	北京市西城区德外大街 4 号	网　　址	http://www.hep.edu.cn
邮政编码	100120		http://www.hep.com.cn
印　　刷	北京中科印刷有限公司	网上订购	http://www.landraco.com
开　　本	889mm×1194mm　1/16		http://www.landraco.com.cn
印　　张	9.25		
插　　页	2	版　　次	2012 年 5 月第 1 版
字　　数	330 千字	印　　次	2012 年 5 月第 1 次印刷
购书热线	010 - 58581118	定　　价	24.00 元

医学教育改革系列教材编委会

《口腔科学》编委会

主　编　孙　正

编　委（以姓氏拼音为序）

柏景坪　韩正学　侯晓玫　黄　欣　贾海鸥

刘静明　单兆臣　孙　正　王冬青　邢汝东

杨晓江

Foreword

Global developments in medicine and health shape trends in medical education. And in China education reform has become an important focus as the country strives to meet the basic requirements for developing a medical education system that meets international standards. Significant medical developments abroad are now being incorporated into the education of both domestic and international medical students in China, which includes students from Hong Kong, Macao and Taiwan that are taught through mandarin Chinese as well as students from a variety of other regions that are taught through the English language. This latter group creates higher demands for both schools and teachers.

Unfortunately there is no consensus as to how to improve the level and quality of education for these students or even as to which English language materials should be used. Some teachers prefer to directly use original English language materials, while others make use of Chinese medical textbooks with the help of English language medical notes. The lack of consensus has emerged from the lack of English language medical textbooks based on the characteristics of modern medical education in China.

In fact, most Chinese teachers involved in medical education have already attained an adequate level of English language usage. However, English language medical textbooks that reflect the culture of the teachers would in fact make it easier for these teachers to complete the task at hand and would improve the level and quality of medical education for international students. In addition, these texts could be used to improve the English language level of the medical students taught in Chinese. This is the purpose behind the compilation and publishing of this set of English language medical education textbooks.

The editors in chief are mainly experts in medicine from Capital Medical University (CCMU). The editorial board members are mainly teachers of a variety of subjects from CCMU. In addition, teachers with rich teaching experience in other medical schools are also called upon to help create this set of textbooks. And finally some excellent scholars are invited to participate as final arbiters for some of the materials.

The total package of English medical education textbooks includes 63 books. Each textbook conforms to five standards according to their grounding in science; adherence to a system; basic theory, concepts and skills elucidated; simplicity and practicality. This has enabled the creation of a series of English language textbooks that adheres to the characteristics and customs of Chinese medical education. The complete set of textbooks conforms to an overall design and uniform style in regards to covers, colors, and graphics. Each chapter contains learning objectives, core concepts, an introduction, a body, a summary, questions and references that together serve as a scaffold for both teachers and students.

The complete set of English language medical education textbooks is designed for teaching overseas undergraduate clinical medicine students (six years), and can also serve as reference textbooks for bilingual teaching and learning for 5-year, 7-year and 8-year programs in clinical medicine.

We would like to thank the chief arbiters, chief editors and general editors for their arduous labor in the writing of each chapter. We would also like to acknowledge all the contributors. Finally, we would like to acknowledge Higher Education Press. They have all provided valuable support during the many weekends and evening hours of work that were necessary for completing this endeavor.

President of Capital Medical University
Director of English Textbook Compiling Commission
Zhaofeng Lu
August 1st, 2011

Preface

This textbook is written for medical students as an introduction to the study of anatomy of the teeth and oral cavity, common diseases in the teeth and oral and maxillofacial region. The book includes 12 chapters: introduction to dental and oral anatomy, cariology and endodontics, periodontal diseases, recurrent aphthous stomatitis, intraoral local anesthesia, dental extractions, infection and inflammation of the tooth and jaws, oral and maxillofacial injuries, temporomandibular disorders, maxillofacial pathology, geriatric dentistry, oral manifestations of systemic diseases.

The text is written in brief and do not involve all aspects of the dentistry because it is mainly intended for medical students. But it can also be used as a reference for dental students in the process of bilingual teaching. The aim of this book is to provide the students with the general idea and understanding of dentistry. One of the features of the book is that each chapter lists objectives, key concepts and introduction at the beginning, summary and questions at the end, which enhances its usefulness to both teachers and students. It is hoped this introductory book will help gain general knowledge about dentistry.

Professor and Dean
School of Stomatology
Capital Medical University
Zheng Sun
March, 2012

Contributors

Jingping Bai 柏景坪
School of Stomatology
Capital Medical University, Beijing, China

Zhengxue Han 韩正学
School of Stomatology
Capital Medical University, Beijing, China

Xiaomei Hou 侯晓玫
School of Stomatology
Capital Medical University, Beijing, China

Xin Huang 黄欣
School of Stomatology
Capital Medical University, Beijing, China

Haiou Jia 贾海鸥
School of Stomatology
Capital Medical University, Beijing, China

Jingming Liu 刘静明
School of Stomatology
Capital Medical University, Beijing, China

Zhaochen Shan 单兆臣
School of Stomatology
Capital Medical University, Beijing, China

Zheng Sun 孙正
School of Stomatology
Capital Medical University, Beijing, China

Dongqing Wang 王冬青
School of Stomatology
Capital Medical University, Beijing, China

Rudong Xing 邢汝东
School of Stomatology
Capital Medical University, Beijing, China

Xiaojiang Yang 杨晓江
School of Stomatology
Capital Medical University, Beijing, China

CONTENTS

Chapter 1

Introduction to Dental and Oral Anatomy

▪ Objectives

Provide a comprehensive introduction of dental anatomy.

Identify two areas of the oral cavity, the boundaries of the oral vestibule, and the boundaries of the oral cavity proper.

Describe each structure of the oral cavity as to location, color, size, and/or shape.

Define the terms noted in boldface.

Complete the worksheet at the end of the chapter.

Perform the clinical applications at the end of the chapter.

▪ Key Concepts

Dental anatomy or anatomy of teeth is a field of anatomy dedicated to the study of human tooth structures.

▪ Introduction

Dental anatomy is defined here as, but is not limited to, the study of the development, morphology, function, and identity of each of the teeth in the human dentitions, as well as the way in which the teeth relate in shape, form, structure, color, and function to the other teeth in the same dental arch and to the teeth in the opposing arch. Thus, the study of dental anatomy, physiology, and occlusion provides one of the basic components of the skills needed to practice all phases of dentistry.

The application of dental anatomy to clinical practice can be envisioned in Figure 1-1 A where a disturbance of enamel formation has resulted in esthetic, psychological, and periodontal problems that may be corrected by an appropriate restorative dental treatment such as that illustrated in Figure 1-1 B. The practitioner has to have knowledge of the morphology, occlusion, esthetics, phonetics, and functions of these teeth to undertake such treatment.

1.1 Dental Anatomy

1.1.1 Formation of the Dentitions (Overview)

Humans have two sets of teeth in their lifetime. The first set of teeth to be seen in the mouth is the **primary** or **deciduous** dentition, which begins to form prenatally at about 14 weeks in utero and is completed postnatally at about 3 years of age. In the absence of congenital disorders, dental disease, or trauma, the first teeth in this dentition begin to appear in the oral cavity at the mean age of 6, and the last emerge at a mean age of 28 ± 4 months. The deciduous dentition remains intact (barring loss from dental caries or trauma) until the child is about 6 years of age. At about that time the first **succedaneous** or **permanent** teeth begin to emerge into the mouth. The emergence of these teeth begins the **transition** or **mixed dentition period** in which there is a mixture of deciduous and succedaneous teeth present. The transition period lasts from about 6 to 12 years of age and ends when all the deciduous teeth have been shed. At that time the permanent dentition period begins. Thus, the transition from the primary dentition to the permanent dentition begins with the emergence of the first permanent molars, shedding of the deciduous incisors, and emergence of the permanent incisors. The mixed dentition period is often a difficult time for the young child because of habits, missing teeth, teeth of different colors and hues, crowding of the teeth, and malposed teeth.

The permanent, or succedaneous, teeth replace the exfoliated deciduous teeth in a sequence of eruption that exhibits some variance.

After the shedding of the deciduous canines and molars, emergence of the permanent canines and premolars, and emergence of the second permanent molars, the permanent dentition is completed (including the roots) at about 14 to 15 years of age, except for the third molars, which are completed at 18 to 25 years of age. In effect, the duration of the permanent dentition period is 12+ years. The completed permanent dentition consists of 32 teeth if none are congenitally missing, which may be the case.

1.1.2 Nomenclature

The first step in understanding dental anatomy is to learn the nomenclature, or the system of names,

used to describe or classify the material included in the subject. When a significant term is used for the first time here, it is emphasized in bold. Additional terms will be discussed as needed in subsequent chapters.

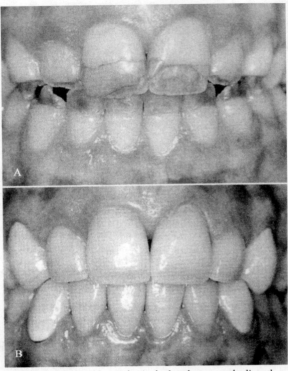

Figure 1-1 A. Chronological developmental disorder involving all the anterior teeth. **B.** Illustration of restored teeth just after completion, taking in account esthetics, occlusion, and periodontal health. Note that the gingival response is not yet resolved
(From Ash MM, Ramfjord S. Occlusion. 4ᵗʰ ed. Philadelphia: Saunders, 1995.)

The term **mandibular** refers to the lower jaw, or mandible. The term **maxillary** refers to the upper jaw, or maxilla. When more than one name is used in the literature to describe something, the two most commonly used names will be used initially. After that they may be combined or used separately as consistent with the literature of a particular specialty of dentistry, for example, **primary** or **deciduous dentition**, **permanent** or **succedaneous dentition**. A good case may be made for the use of both terms. By dictionary definition, the term **primary** can mean "constituting or belonging to the first stage in any process." The term **deciduous** can mean "not permanent, transitory." The same unabridged dictionary refers the reader from the definition of **deciduous**

tooth to milk tooth, which is defined as "one of the temporary teeth of a mammal that are replaced by permanent teeth, also called **baby tooth, deciduous tooth**." The term **primary** can indicate a first dentition and the term **deciduous** can indicate that the first dentition is not permanent, but not unimportant. The term **succedaneous** can be used to describe a successor dentition and does not suggest permanence, whereas the term **permanent** suggests a permanent dentition, which may not be the case due to dental caries, periodontal diseases, and trauma. All four of these descriptive terms appear in the professional literature.

1.1.3 Formulae for Mammalian Teeth

The denomination and number of all mammalian teeth are expressed by formulae that are used to differentiate the human dentitions from those of other species. The denomination of each tooth is often represented by the initial letter in its name (e.g. I for incisor, C for canine, P for premolar, M for molar). Each letter is followed by a horizontal line and the number for each type of tooth is placed above the line for the maxilla (upper jaw) and below the line for the mandible (lower jaw). The formulae include one side only, with the number of teeth in each jaw being the same for humans.

The dental formula for the primary/deciduous teeth in humans is as follows:

$$I\frac{2}{2}C\frac{1}{1}M\frac{2}{2}=10$$

This formula should be read as: incisors, two maxillary and two mandibular; canines, one maxillary and one mandibular; molar, two maxillary and two mandibular—or 10 altogether on one side, right or left (Figure 1-2 A).

A dental formula for the permanent human dentition is as follows:

$$I\frac{2}{2}C\frac{1}{1}P\frac{2}{2}M\frac{3}{3}=16$$

Premolars have now been added to the formula, two maxillary and two mandibular, and a third molar has been added, one maxillary and one mandibular (Figure1-2 B).

Systems for scoring key morphological traits of the permanent dentition that are used for anthropological studies are not described here. However, a few of the morphological traits that are used in anthropological studies are considered in the following chapters (e.g. shoveling, Carabelli's trait, enamel extensions, and peg-shaped incisors). Some anthropologists use di_1, di_2, dc, dm_1, and dm_2 notations for the deciduous dentition and I_1, I_2, C, P_2, M_1, M_2, and M_3 for the permanent teeth. These notations are generally limited to anthropological tables because of keyboard incompatibility.

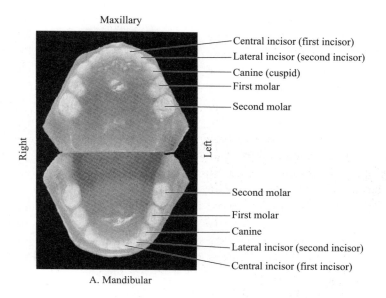

Maxillary

- Central incisor (first incisor)
- Lateral incisor (second incisor)
- Canine (cuspid)
- First molar
- Second molar

Right / Left

- Second molar
- First molar
- Canine
- Lateral incisor (second incisor)
- Central incisor (first incisor)

A. Mandibular

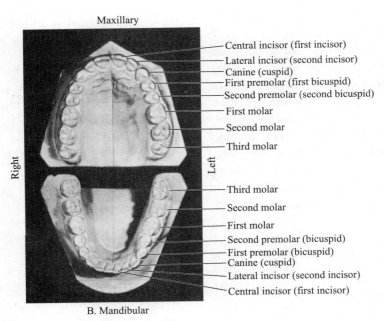

Figure 1-2 A. Casts of deciduous, or primary, dentition. **B.** Casts of permanent dentition
(A from Berkovitz BK, Holland GR, Moxham BJ. Oral anatomy, histology and embryology. 3rd ed. St. Louis: Mosby, 2002.)

1.1.4 Tooth Numbering Systems

In clinical practice some "shorthand" system of tooth notation is necessary for recording data. There are several systems in use in the world, but only a few are considered here. In 1947 a committee of the American Dental Association (ADA) recommended the symbolic (Zsigmondy/Palmer) system as the numbering method of choice. However, because of difficulties with keyboard notation of the symbolic notation system, the ADA in 1968 officially recommended the "universal" numbering system. Because of some limitations and lack of widespread use internationally, recommendations for a change sometimes are made.

The **universal** system of notation for the primary dentition uses uppercase letters for each of the primary teeth: For the maxillary teeth, beginning with the right second molar, letters A through J, and for the mandibular teeth, letters K through T, beginning with the left mandibular second molar. The universal system notation for the entire primary dentition is as follows:

Midsagittal plane

Right   A B C D E | F G H I J   Left
          T S R Q P | O N M L K

The **symbolic** system for the permanent dentition was introduced by Adolph Zsigmondy of Vienna is 1861 and then modified for the primary dentition in 1874. Independently, Palmer also published the symbolic system in 1870. The symbolic system is most often referred to as the **Palmer notation system** in the United States and less frequently as the **Zsigmondy/Palmer notation system**. In this system the arches are divided into quadrants with the entire dentition being notated as follows:

E D C B A | A B C D E
E D C B A | A B C D E

Thus, for a single tooth such as the maxillary right central incisor the designation is A| . For the mandibular left central incisor, the notation is given as |A . This numbering system presents difficulty when as appropriate font is not available for keyboard recording of Zsigmondy/Palmer symbolic notations. For simplification this symbolic notation is often designated as Palmer's dental notation rather than Zsigmondy/Palmer notation.

In the **universal notation system** for the permanent dentition, the maxillary teeth are numbered from 1 through 16, beginning with the right third molar. Beginning with the mandibular left third molar, the teeth are numbered 17 through 32. Thus, the right maxillary first molar is designated as 3, the maxillary left central incisor as 9, and the right mandibular first molar as 30. The following universal notation designates the entire permanent dentition.

1	2	3	4	5	6	7	8	9	10	11	12	13	14	15	16
32	31	30	29	28	27	26	25	24	23	22	21	20	19	18	17

The Zsigmondy/Palmer notation for the permanent dentition is a four-quadrant symbolic system in which, beginning with the central incisors, the teeth are numbered 1 through 8 (or more) in each arch. For example, the right maxillary first molar is designated as 6⌋, and the left mandibular central incisor as ⌈1 . The Palmer notation for the entire permanent dentition is as follows:

8	7	6	5	4	3	2	1	1	2	3	4	5	6	7	8
8	7	6	5	4	3	2	1	1	2	3	4	5	6	7	8

Viktor Haderup of Denmark in 1891 devised a variant of the eight-tooth quadrant system in which plus(+) and minus (−) were used to differentiate between upper and lower quadrants and between right and left quadrants; in other words, +1 indicates the upper left central incisor and 1- indicates the lower right central incisor. Primary teeth were numbered as follows: upper right, 05+ to 01+; lower left, −01 to −05. This system is still taught in Denmark.

The universal system is acceptable to computer language, whereas the Palmer notation is generally incompatible with computers and word processing systems. Each tooth in the universal system is designated with a unique number, which leads to less confusion than with the Palmer notation.

A two-digit system proposed by Federation Dentaire Internationale (FDI) for both the primary and permanent dentitions has been adopted by the World Health Organization and accepted by other organizations such as the international association for dental research. The FDI system of tooth notation is as follows.

For the primary teeth:

	Upper right				Upper left			
55	54	53	52	51	61	62	63	64	65
85	84	83	82	81	71	72	73	74	75
	Lower right				Lower left			

Numeral 5 indicates the maxillary right side, and 6 indicates the maxillary left side. The second number of the two-digit number is the tooth number for each side. The number 8 indicates the mandibular right side, and the number 7 indicates the mandibular left side. The second number of the two-digit system is the tooth number. Thus, for example

the number 51 refers to **the maxillary right central incisor.**

For the permanent teeth:

	Upper right						Upper left					
18	17	16	15	14	13	12	11	21	22	23	24	25	26	27	28
48	47	46	45	44	43	42	41	31	32	33	34	35	36	37	38
	Lower right						Lower left					

Thus, as in the two-digit FDI system for the primary dentition, the first digit indicates the quadrant: 1 to 4 for the permanent dentition and 5 to 8 for the primary dentition. The second digit indicates the tooth within a quadrant: 1 to 8 for the permanent teeth and 1 to 5 for the primary teeth. For example, the permanent upper right central incisor is 11 (pronounced "one one," not "eleven").

1.1.5 The Crown and Root

Each tooth has a crown and root portion. The crown is covered with enamel, and the root portion is covered with cementum. The crown and root join at the cementoenamel junction (CEJ). This junction, also called the **cervical line** (Figure 1-3), is plainly visible on a specimen tooth. The main bulk of the tooth is composed of dentin, which is clear in a cross section of the tooth. This cross section displays a pulp chamber and a pulp canal, which normally contain the pulp tissue. The pulp chamber is in the crown portion mainly, and the pulp canal is in the root (Figure 1-4). The spaces are continuous with each other and are spoken of collectively as the **pulp cavity.**

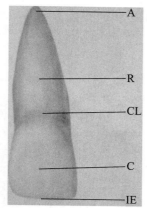

**Figure 1-3 Maxillary central incisor
(facial aspect)**
A: Apex of root; R: root; CL: cervical line;
C: crown; IE: incisal edge

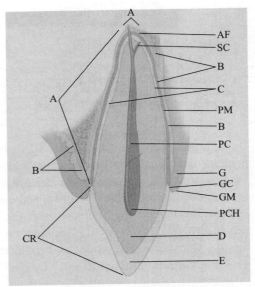
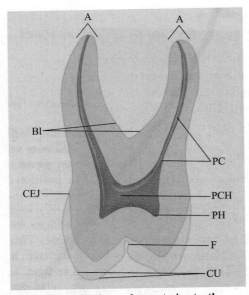

Figure 1-4   **Schematic drawings of longitudinal sections of an anterior and a posterior tooth**

A. anterior tooth. A: apex; AF: apical foramen; GM: gingival margin; SC: supplementary canal; B: bone; C: cementum; PM: periodontal ligament; PC: pulp canal; G: gingiva; GC: gingival crevice; PCH: pulp chamber; D: dentin; E: enamel; CR: crown; B. Posterior tooth. A: apices; PH: pulp horn; F: fissure; CU: cusp; CEJ: cementoenamel junction; BI: bifurcation of roots

The four tooth tissues are enamel, cementum, dentin and pulp. The first three are known as **hard tissues**, the last as **soft tissue**. The pulp tissue furnishes the blood and nerve supply to the tooth. The tissues of the teeth must be considered in relation to the other tissues of the orofacial structures (Figures 1-5 and 1-6) if the physiology of the teeth is to be understood.

The crown of an incisor tooth may have an incisal ridge or edge, as in the central and lateral incisors; a single cusp, as in the canines; or two or more cusps, as on premolars and molars. Incisal ridges and cusps form the cutting surfaces on tooth crowns.

The root portion of the tooth may be single, with one apex or terminal end, as usually found in anterior teeth and some of the premolars; or multiple, with a bifurcation or trifurcation dividing the root portion into two or more extensions or roots with their apices or terminal ends, as found on all molars and in some premolars.

The root portion of the tooth is firmly fixed in the bony process of the jaw, so that each tooth is held in its position relative to the others in the dental arch. That portion of the jaw serving as support for the tooth is called the **alveolar process.** The bone of the tooth socket is called the *alveolus* (plural, alveoli) (Figure 1-7).

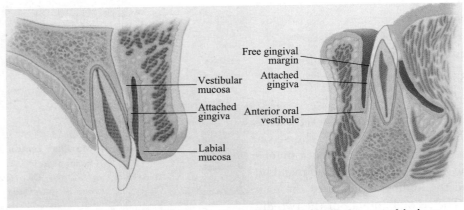

Figure 1-5   **Sagittal sections through the maxillary and mandibular central incisors**

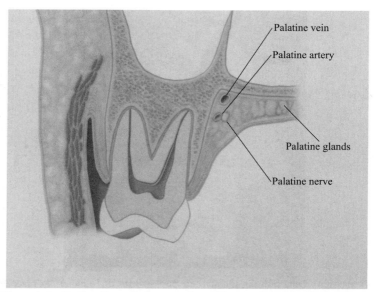

Figure 1-6   Section through the second maxillary molar and adjacent tissues

The crown portion is never covered by bone tissue after it is fully erupted, but it is partly covered at the cervical third in young adults by soft tissue of the mouth known as the *gingiva* or *gingival tissue*, or "gums". In some persons, all of the enamel and frequently some cervical cementum may not be covered by the gingiva.

1. 1. 5. 1   Surfaces and ridges

The crowns of the incisors and canines have four surfaces and a ridge, and the crowns of the premolars and molars have five surfaces. The surfaces are named according to their positions and uses (Figure 1-8). In the incisors and canines, the surfaces toward the lips are called **labial surfaces**; in the premolars and molars, those facing the cheek are the **buccal surfaces**. When labial and buccal surfaces are spoken of collectively, they are called **facial surfaces**. All surfaces facing toward the tongue are called **lingual surfaces**. The surfaces of the premolars and molars that come in contact (occlusion) with those in the opposite jaw during the act of closure are called **occlusal surfaces**. These are called **incisal surfaces** with respect to incisors and canines.

The surfaces of the teeth facing toward adjoining teeth in the same dental arch are called **proximal** or **proximate surfaces**. The proximal surfaces may be called either **mesial** or **distal**. These terms have special reference to the position of the surface relative to the median line of the face. This line is drawn vertically through the center of the face, passing between the central incisors at their point of contact with each other in both the maxilla and the mandible. Those proximal surfaces that, following the curve of the arch, are faced toward the median line are called **mesial surfaces**, and those most distant from the median line are called **distal surfaces**.

Four teeth have mesial surfaces that contact each other: the **maxillary** and **mandibular central incisors**. In all other instances, the mesial surface of one tooth contacts the distal surface of its neighbor, except for the distal surfaces of third molars of permanent teeth and distal surfaces of second molars in deciduous teeth, which have no teeth distal to them. The area of the mesial or distal surface of a tooth that touches its neighbor in the arch is called the **contact area**.

Central and lateral incisors and canines as a group are called **anterior teeth**; premolars and molars as a group, **posterior teeth**.

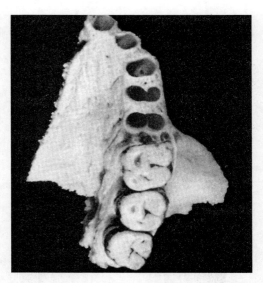

Figure 1-7   Left maxillary bone showing the alveolar process with three molars in place and the alveoli of the central incisor, lateral incisor, canine, and first and second premolars

Note the opening at the bottom of the canine alveolus, an opening that accommodates the nutrient blood and nerve supply to the tooth in life. Although they do not show up in the photograph, the other alveoli present the same arrangement

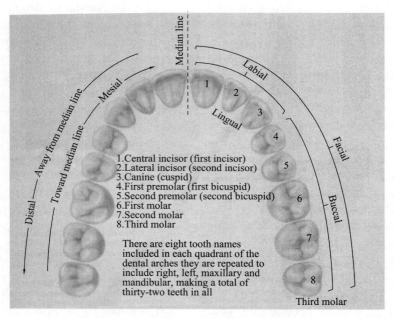

1.Central incisor (first incisor)
2.Lateral incisor (second incisor)
3.Canine (cuspid)
4.First premolar (first bicuspid)
5.Second premolar (second bicuspid)
6.First molar
7.Second molar
8.Third molar

There are eight tooth names included in each quadrant of the dental arches they are repeated to include right, left, maxillary and mandibular, making a total of thirty-two teeth in all

Figure 1-8   Application of nomenclature

Tooth numbers 1 to 8 indicating left maxillary teeth. Tooth surfaces related to the tongue (lingual), cheek (buccal), lips (labial), and face (facial), apply to four quadrants and the upper left quadrant. The teeth or their parts or surfaces may be described as being away from the midline (distal) or toward the midline (mesial)

1.1.5.2   Other landmarks

To study an individual tooth intelligently, one should recognize all landmarks of importance by name. Therefore, at this point it is necessary to become familiar with additional terms, such as the following:

Cusp	triangular ridge	developmental groove
Tubercle	transverse ridge	supplemental groove
Cingulum	oblique ridge	pit
Ridge	fossa	lobe
Marginal	ridge	sulcus

A **cusp** is an elevation or mound on the crown

portion of a tooth making up a divisional part of the occlusal surface(Figures 1-4 and 1-9).

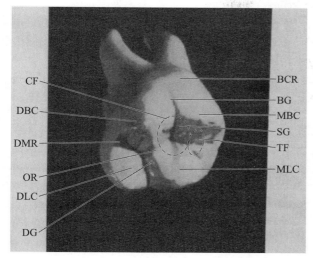

Figure 1-9   Some Landmarks on the maxillary first molar
BCR, buccocervical ridge; BG, buccal groove; MBC, mesiobuccal cusp; SG supplemental groove; TF, triangular fossa; MLC, mesiolingual cusp; DG, developmental groove; DLC distolingual cusp; OR, oblique ridge; DMR, distal marginal ridge; DBC, distobuccal cusp; CF, central fossa

A **tubercle** is a smaller elevation on some portion of the crown produced by an extra formation of enamel. These are deviations from the typical form.

A **cingulum** (Latin word for "girdle")is the lingual lobe of an anterior tooth. It makes up the bulk of the cervical third of the lingual surface. Its convexity mesiodistally resembles a girdle encircling the lingual surface at the cervical third (Figure 1-10).

A **ridge** is any linear elevation on the surface of a tooth and is named according to its location (e. g. buccal ridge, incisal ridge, marginal ridge).

Marginal ridges are those rounded borders of the enamel that form the mesial and distal margins of the occlusal surfaces of premolars and molars and the mesial and distal margins of the lingual surfaces of the incisors and canines(Figures 1-10 A, and 1-11).

Triangular ridges descend from the tips of the cusps of molars and premolars toward the central part of the occlusal surfaces. They are so named because the slopes of each side of the ridge are inclined to resemble two sides of a triangle(Figures 1-11 B and C, and 1-12). They are named after the cusps to which they belong, for example, the triangular ridge of the buccal cusp of the maxillary first premolar.

When a buccal and a lingual triangular ridge join, they form a **transverse ridge**. A transverse ridge is the union of two triangular ridges crossing transversely the surface of a posterior tooth (Figure 1-11 B and C).

The **oblique ridge** is a ridge crossing obliquely the occlusal surfaces of maxillary molars and formed by the union of the triangular ridge of the distobuccal cusp and the distal cusp ridge of the mesiolingual cusp(Figure 1-9).

A **fossa** is an irregular depression or concavity. **Lingual fossae** are on the lingual surface of incisors (Figure 1-10).

Central fossae are on the occlusal surface of molars. They are formed by the convergence of ridges terminating at a central point in the bottom of the depression where there is a junction of grooves (Figure 1-12). **Triangular fossae** are found on molars and premolars on the occlusal surfaces mesial or distal to marginal ridges (Figure 1-9). They are sometimes found on the lingual surfaces of maxillary incisors at the edge of the lingual fossae where the marginal ridges and the cingulum meet.

A **sulcus** is a long depression or valley in the surface of a tooth between ridges and cusps, the inclines of which meet at an angle. A sulcus has a developmental groove at the junction of its inclines. (The term **sulcus** should not be confused with the term **groove**).

A **developmental groove** is a shallow groove or line between the primary parts of the crown or root. A **supplemental groove**, less distinct, is also a shallow linear depression on the surface of a tooth, but it is supplemental to a developmental groove and does not mark the junction of primary parts. **Buccal** and **lingual grooves** are developmental grooves found on the buccal and lingual surfaces of posterior teeth (Figures 1-9 and 1-12).

Pits are small pinpoint depressions located at the junction of developmental grooves or at terminals of those grooves. For instance, central pit is a term used to describe a landmark in the central fossa of molars where developmental grooves join (Figure 1-11 C).

A **lobe** is one of the primary sections of formation in the development of the crown. Cusps and mamelons are representative of lobes. A **mamelon** is any one of the three rounded protuberances found on the incisal ridges of newly erupted incisor teeth (Figure 1-10 B).

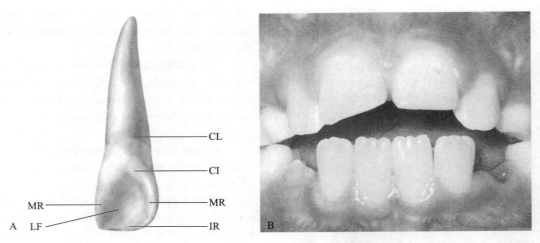

Figure 1-10 A. Maxillary right central incisor (lingual aspect). **B.** Mamelons on erupting, noncontacting central incisors
CL, cervical line; CI, cingulum (also called the linguocervical ridge); MR, marginal ridge; IR, incisal ridge; LF, lingual fossa
(B from Bath-Balogh M, Fehrenbach MJ. Illustrated dental embryology, histology, and anatomy. 2nd ed. St. Louis:Saunders,2006.)

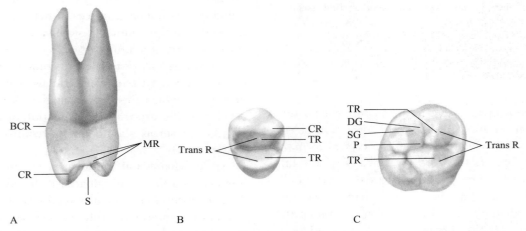

Figure 1-11 A. Mesial view of a maxillary right first premolar. **B.** Occlusal view of maxillary right first premolar.
C. Occlusal view of a maxillary right first molar
MR, marginal ridge; S, sulcus traversing occlusal surface; CR, cusp ridge; BCR, buccocervical ridge; TR, triangular ridges;
Trans R, transverse ridge, formed by two triangular ridges that cross the tooth transversely; P, pit formed by junction of developmental grooves; SG, supplemental groove; DG, developmental groove

The **roots** of the teeth may be single or multiple. Both maxillary and mandibular anterior teeth have only one root each. Mandibular first and second premolars and the maxillary second premolar are single rooted, but the maxillary first premolar has two roots in most cases, one buccal and one lingual. Maxillary molars have three roots, one mesiobuccal, one distobuccal, and one lingual. Mandibular molars have two roots, one mesial and one distal. It must be understood that description in anatomy can never follow a hard-and-fast rule. Variations frequently occur. This is especially true regarding tooth roots, for example, facial and lingual roots of the mandibu-

lar canine.

1. 1. 5. 3   Division into thirds, line angles, and point angles

For purposes of description, the crowns and roots of teeth have been divided into thirds, and junctions of the crown surfaces are described as line angles and point angles. Actually, there are no angles or points or plane surfaces on the teeth anywhere except those that appear from wear (e. g. **attrition, abrasion**) or from accidental fracture. Line angle and point angle are used only as descriptive terms to indicate a location.

When the surfaces of the crown and root portions are divided into thirds, these thirds are named according to their location. Looking at the tooth from the labial or buccal aspect, we see that the crown and root may be divided into thirds from the incisal or occlusal surface of the crown to the apex of the root (Figure 1-13). The crown is divided into an incisal or occlusal third, a middle third, and a cervical third. The root is divided into a cervical third, a middle third, and an apical third.

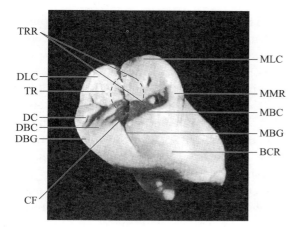

Figure 1-12　Mandibular right first molar

MLC, mesiolingual cusp; MMR, mesial marginal ridge; MBC, mesiobuccal cusp; MBG, mesiobuccal groove; BCR, buccocervical ridge; CF, central fossa; DBG, distobuccal groove; DBC, distobuccal cusp; DC, distal cusp; TR, triangular ridge; DLC, distolingual cusp; TRR, transverse ridge

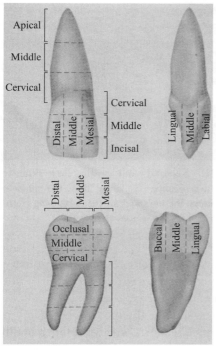

Figure 1-13　Division into thirds

The crown may be divided into thirds in three directions: inciso- or occlusocervically, mesiodistally, or labio- or buccolingually. Mesiodistally, it is divided into the mesial, middle, and distal thirds. Labio- or buccolingually it is divided into labial or buccal, middle, and lingual thirds. Each of the five surfaces of a crown may be so divided. There will be one middle third and two other thirds, which are named according to their location, for example, cervical, occlusal, mesial, lingual.

A **line angle** is formed by the junction of two surfaces and derives its name from the combination of the two surfaces that join. For instance, on an anterior tooth, the junction of the mesial and labial surfaces is called the **mesiolabial line angle**.

The line angles of the **anterior teeth** (Figure 1-14 A) are as follows:

Mesiolabial	distolabial
Distolingual	labioincisal
Mesiolingual	linguoincisal

Because the mesial and distal incisal angles of anterior teeth are rounded, **mesioincisal line angles** and **distoincisal line angles** are usually considered nonexistent. They are spoken of as mesial and distal incisal angles only.

The line angles of the **posterior teeth** (Figure 1-14 B) are as follows:

Mesiobuccal	distobuccal
Mesiolingual	distolingual
Mesio-occlusal	disto-occlusal
Bucco-occlusal	linguo-occlusal

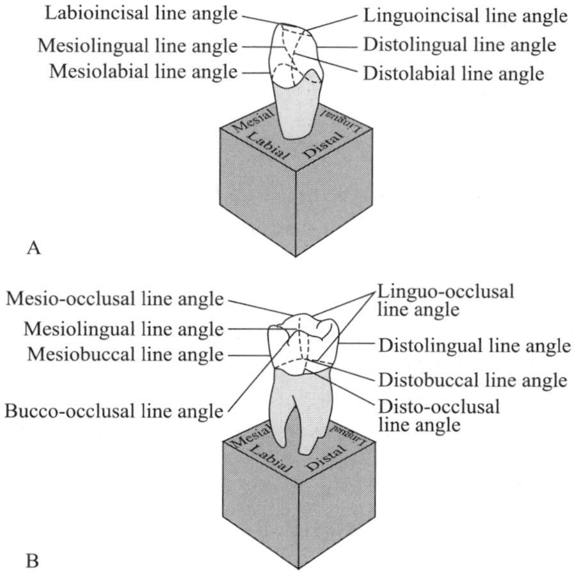

Labioincisal line angle — Linguoincisal line angle
Mesiolingual line angle — Distolingual line angle
Mesiolabial line angle — Distolabial line angle

A

Mesio-occlusal line angle — Linguo-occlusal line angle
Mesiolingual line angle — Distolingual line angle
Mesiobuccal line angle — Distobuccal line angle
Bucco-occlusal line angle — Disto-occlusal line angle

B

Figure 1-14　Line angles
A. Anterior teeth. **B.** Posterior teeth

A **point angle** is formed by the junction of three surfaces. The point angle also derives its name from the combination of the names of the surfaces forming it. For example, the junction of the mesial, buccal, and occlusal surfaces of a molar is called the **mesio-bucco-occlusal point angle.**

The point angles of the **anterior teeth** are (Figure 1-15 A):

Mesiolabioincisal   distolabioincisal
Mesiolinguoincisal   distolinguoincisal

The point angles of the **posterior teeth** are (Figure 1-15 B):

Mesiobucco-occlusal   mesiolinguo-occlusal
Distobucco-occlusal   distolinguo-occlusal

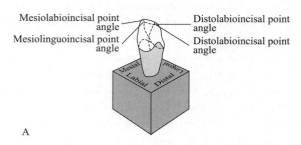

A

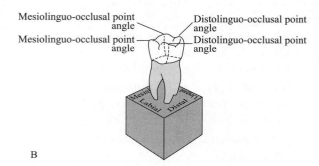

B

Figure 1-15 A. Point angles on anterior teeth.
B. Point angles on posterior teeth

1.1.6   Tooth Drawing and Carving

The subject of drawing and carving of teeth is being introduced at this point because it has been found through experience that a laboratory course in tooth morphology (dissection, drawing, and carving) should be carried on simultaneously with lectures and reference work on the subject of dental anatomy. Illustrations and instruction in tooth form drawing and carving, however, are not included here.

1.1.7   The Dentitions

The human dentitions are usually categorized as being primary, mixed (transitional), and permanent

dentitions. The transition from the primary/deciduous dentition to the permanent dentition is of particular interest because of changes that may herald the onset of malocclusion and provide for its interception and correction. Thus of importance for the practitioner are the interactions between the morphogenesis of the teeth, development of the dentition, and growth of the craniofacial complex.

1.1.7.1   Prenatal/perinatal/postnatal development

The first indication of tooth formation occurs as early as the sixth week of prenatal life when the jaws have assumed their initial shape; however, at this time the jaws are rather small compared with the large brain case and orbits. The lower face height is small compared with the neurocranium (Figure 1-16). The mandibular arch is larger than the maxillary arch, and the vertical dimensions of the jaws are but little developed. When the jaws close at this stage in the development of the dentition, they make contact with the tongue, which in turn makes contact with the cheeks. The shape of the prenatal head varies considerably, but the relative difference between the brain case, orbits, and lower face height remains the same. All stages of tooth formation fill both jaws during this stage of development.

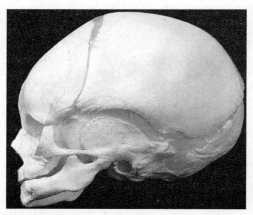

Figure 1-16   Neonatal skull showing large brain case and orbits; the neurocranium is larger than the splanchnocranium, which contains the jaws and all the developing teeth
(From Avery JK, Chiego Jr DJ. Essentials of oral histology and embryology. 3rd ed. St, Louis: Mosby 2006.)

1.1.7.2   Development of the primary dentition

Considerable growth follows birth in the neurocranium and splanchnocranium. Usually at birth, no teeth are visible in the mouth; however, occasionally, infants are born with erupted mandibular incisors. Development of both primary and permanent teeth continues in this period, and jaw growth follows the need for additional space posteriorly for additional teeth. In addition the alveolar bone height increases to accommodate the increasing length of the teeth. However, growth of the anterior parts of the jaws is limited after about the first year of postnatal life.

1. 1. 7. 3   Sequence of emergence of primary teeth

The predominant sequence of eruption of the primary teeth in the individual jaw is central incisor, lateral incisor, first molar, canine, and second molar. Variations in that order may be the result of reversals of central and lateral incisors or first molar and lateral incisor, or eruption of two teeth at the same time.

Investigations of the chronology of emergence of primary teeth in different racial and ethnic groups show considerable variation, and little information is available on tooth formation in populations of nonwhite/non-european ancestry. World population differences in tooth standards suggest that patterned differences may exist that in fact are not large. Tooth size, morphology, and formation are highly inheritable characteristics. Few definitive correlations exist between primary tooth emergence and other physiological parameters such as skeletal maturation, size, and sex.

1. 1. 7. 4   Emergence of the primary teeth

At about 8 (6 to 10) months of age, the mandibular central incisors emerge through the alveolar gingiva, followed by the other anterior teeth, so that by about 13 to 16 months, all eight primary incisors have erupted (see Table 1-1). Then the first primary molars emerge by about 16 months of age and make contact with opposing teeth several months later, before the canines have fully erupted. Passage through the alveolar crest (Figure 1-17) occurs when approximately two thirds of the root is formed, followed by emergences through the alveolar gingiva into the oral cavity when about three fourths of the root is completed. The emergence data are consistent with those of Smith.

Table 1-1 Chronology of primary teeth

Tooth	First evidence of calcification (weeks in utero)	Crown completed (months)	Eruption (months)	Root completed (years)
i1	14(13 – 16)	1½	10(8 – 12)	1½
i2	16(14⅔ – 16½)	2½	11(9 – 13)	2
c	17(15 – 18)	9	19(16 – 22)	3¼
m1	15½(14½ – 17)	6	16(13 – 19)♂ (14 – 18)♀	2½
m2	19(16 – 23½)	11	29(25 – 33)	3
i1	14(13 – 16)	2½	8(6 – 10)	1½
i2	16(14⅔ –)	3	13(10 – 16)	1½
c	17(16 –)	9	20(17 – 23)	3¼
m1	15½(14½ – 17)	5½	16(14 – 18)	2¼
m2	18(17 – 19½)	10	27(23 – 31)♂ (24 – 30)♀	3

i1, Central incisor; i2, lateral incisor; c, canine; m1, first molar; m2, second molar.

The primary first molars emerge with the maxillary molar tending most often to erupt earlier than the mandibular first molar. Some evidence shows a difference by gender for the first primary molars, but no answer is available for why the first molar has a different pattern of sexual dimorphism.

The primary maxillary canines erupt at about 19 (16 to 22) months (Figure 1-18), and the mandibular canines erupt at 20 (17 to 23) months. The primary second mandibular molar erupts at a mean age of 27 (23 to 31, boys; 24 to 30, girls) months, and the primary maxillary second molar follows at a mean age of 29 (25 to 33±1SD) months. In Figures 1-18, A and B, the first molars are in occlusion.

Neuromuscular development

A mature neuromuscular controlled movement of the mandible requires the presence and articulation of the teeth and proprioceptive input from the periodontium. Thus, the contact of opposing first primary molars is the beginning of the development of occlusion and a neuromuscular substrate for more complex mandibular and tongue functions.

1. 1. 7. 5   Primary dentition

The primary/deciduous dentition is considered

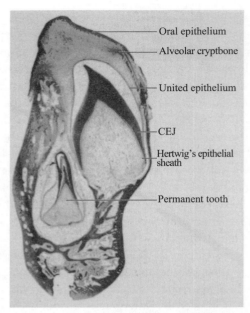

Figure 1-17   Section of mandible in a 9-month-old infant cut through an unerupted primary canine and its permanent successor, which lies lingually and apically to it
The enamel of the primary canine crown is completed and lost because of decalcification. Root formation has begun. CEJ, cementoenamel junction(Modified from Schour I, Noyes HJ. Oral histology and embryology. 8th ed. Philadelphia: Lea & Febiger, 1960.)

to be completed by about 30 months or when the second primary molars are in occlusion (Figure 1-19). The dentition period includes the time when no apparent changes occur intraorally (i. e. from about 30 months to about 6 years of age).

The form of the dental arch remains relatively constant without significant changes in depth or width. A slight increase in the intercanine width occurs about the time the primary incisors are lost, and an increase in size in both jaws in a sagittal direction is consistent with the space needed to accommodate the succedaneous teeth. An increase in the vertical dimension of the facial skeleton occurs as a result of alveolar bone deposition, condyle growth, and deposition of bone at the synchondrosis of the basal part of the occipital bone and sphenoid bones, and at the maxillary suture complex. The splanchnocranium remains small in comparison with the neurocranium. The part of the jaws that contain the primary teeth has almost reached adult width. At the first part of the transition period, which occurs at about age 8, the width of the mandible approximates the width of the neurocranium. The dental arches are complete, and the occlusion of the primary dentition is functional. During this period, attrition is sufficient in many children and is quite observable.

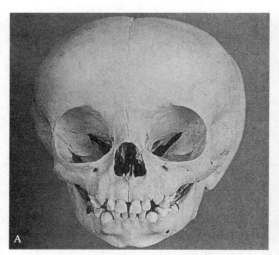
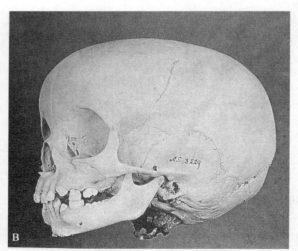

Figure 1-18   Skull of a child about 20 months of age
A. View showing all incisors present and erupting canines. B. Lateral view. First primary molars are in occlusion, mandibular second molars are just emerging opposite the already erupted maxillary molar [Modified from Karl W. Atlas der Zahnheilkunde. Berlin: Verlag von Julius Springer (no publication date available)]

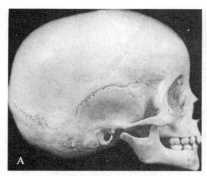
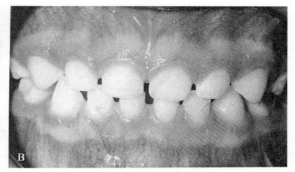

Figure 1-19 A. Skull of child 4 years old with completed primary dentition. **B.** Completed primary dentition
Note the incisal wear (A modified from van der Linden FPGM, Duterloo HS. Development of the human dentition; on atlas. New York; Harper & Row 1976; B from Bird DL, Robinson DS. Modern dental assisting. 9th ed. St. Louis; Saunders 2009.)

1. 1. 7. 6   Transitional (mixed) dentition period

The first transition dentition begins with the emergence and eruption of the mandibular first permanent molars and ends with the loss of the last primary tooth, which usually occurs at about age 11 to 12. The initial phase of the transition period lasts about 2 years, during which time the permanent first molars erupt (Figures 1-20 and 1-21), the primary incisors are shed, and the permanent incisors emerge and erupt into position (Figures 1-22). The permanent teeth do not begin eruptive movements until after the crown is completed. During eruption, the permanent mandibular first molar is guided by the distal surface of the second primary molar. If a distal step in the terminal plane is evident, malocclusion occurs.

1. 1. 7. 7   Loss of primary teeth

The premature loss of primary teeth because of caries has an effect on the development of the permanent dentition and not only may reflect an unfortunate lack of knowledge as to the course of the disease but also establishes a negative attitude about preventing dental caries in the adult dentition. Loss of primary teeth may lead to lack of space for the permanent dentition. It is sometimes assumed by laypersons that the loss of primary teeth, which are sometimes referred to as **baby teeth** or **milk teeth**, is of little consequence because they are only temporary. However, the primary dentition may be in use from age 2 to 7 or older, or about 5 or more years in all. Some of the teeth are in use from 6 months until 12 years of age, or 11. 5 years in all. Thus these primary teeth are in use and contributing to the health and well-being of the individual during the first years of greatest development, physically and mentally.

Premature loss of primary teeth, retention of primary teeth, congenital absence of teeth, dental anomalies, and insufficient space are considered important factors in the initiation and development of an abnormal occlusion. Premature loss of primary teeth from dental neglect is likely to cause a loss of arch length with a consequent tendency for crowding of the permanent dentition.

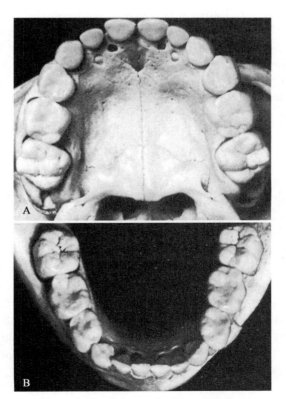

Figure 1-20   Primary dentition with first permanent molars present
A. Maxillary arch. B. Mandibular arch

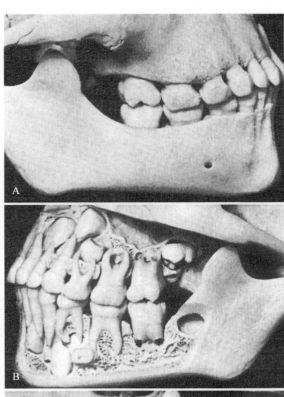

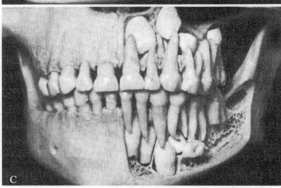

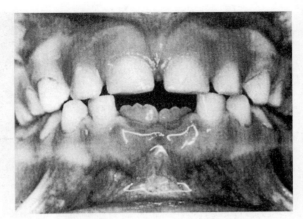

Figure 1-22   Eruption of the permanent central incisors
Note the incisal edges demonstrating mamelons and the width of the emerging incisors

Figure 1-21   Same child as in Figure 1-20
A. Right side. B. Left side showing position of first permanent molars and empty bony crypt of developing second molar lost during preparation of the specimen. C. Front view showing right side with bone covering roots and developing permanent teeth, and left side with developing anterior permanent teeth

1. 1. 7. 8   Permanent dentition

The permanent dentition consisting of 32 teeth is completed from 18 to 25 years of age if the third molar is included.

Apparently there are four or more **centers of formation** (developmental lobes) for each tooth. The formation of each center proceeds until a coalescence of all of them takes place. During this period of odontogenesis, injury to the developing tooth can lead to anomalous morphological features (e. g. peg-shaped lateral incisor). Although no lines of demarcation are found in the dentin to show this development, signs are found on the surfaces of the crowns and roots; these are called **developmental grooves.** Fractures of the teeth occur most commonly along these grooves.

The **follicles** of the developing **incisors** and **canines** are in a position lingual to the deciduous roots (see Figures 1-17 and 1-21).

The developing **premolars**, which eventually take the place of deciduous molars, are within the bifurcation of primary molar roots (Figure 1-23 A and B). The permanent incisors, canines, and premolars are called **succedaneous** teeth because they take the place of their primary predecessors.

The central incisor is the second permanent tooth to emerge into the oral cavity. Eruption time is quite close to that of the first molar (i. e. tooth emergence occurs between 6 and 7 years) (Table 1-2). As with the first molar, at 6 years 50% of individuals have reached the stage considered to be the age of attainment of the stage or, more specifically, the age of emergence for the central incisor. The mandibular permanent teeth tend to erupt before maxillary teeth. The mandibular central incisor usually erupts before the maxillary central incisor (see Figure 1-22) and may erupt simultaneously with or even before the mandibular first molar. The mandibular lateral incisor may erupt along with the central incisor.

Before the permanent central incisor can come into position, the primary central incisor must be exfoliated. This is brought about by the resorption

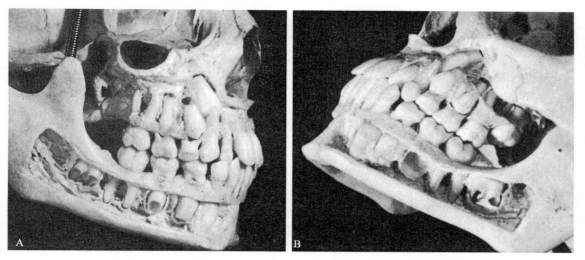

Figure 1-23 A. view of the right side of the skull of a child of **9** to **10** year of age. Note the amount of resorption of the roots of the primary maxillary molars, the relationship of the developing premolars above them, and the open pulp chambers and the pulp canals in the developing mandibular teeth. The roots of the first permanent molars have been completed. **B.** left side. Note the placement of the permanent maxillary canine and second premolar, and the position and stage of development of the maxillary second permanent molar. The bony crypt of the lost mandibular second permanent premolar is in full view. Note the large openings in the roots of the mandibular second permanent molar

of the deciduous roots. The permanent tooth in its follicle attempts to move into the position held by its predecessor. Its influence on the primary root evidently causes resorption of the root, which continues until the primary crown has lost its anchorage, becomes loose, and is finally exfoliated. In the meantime, the permanent tooth has moved occlusally so that when the primary tooth is lost, the permanent one is at the point of eruption and in proper position to succeed its predecessor.

Mandibular lateral incisors erupt very soon after the central incisors, often simultaneously. The **max-**illary central incisors** erupt next in chronological order, and **maxillary lateral incisors** make their appearance about 1 year later (Table 1-2). The **first premolars** follow the maxillary laterals in sequence when the child is about 10 years old; the **mandibular canines** (cuspids) often appear at the same time. The **second premolars** follow during the next year, and then the **maxillary canines** follow. Usually, the second molars come in when the individual is about 12 years of age; they are posterior to the first molars and are commonly called **12-year molars.**

Table 1-2 Chronology of permanent teeth

Tooth		First evidence of calcification	Crown completed (years)	Emergence (Eruption) (years)	Root completed (years)
I1	8, 9	3 – 4 mo	4 – 5	7 – 8	10
I2	7, 10	10 – 12 mo	4 – 5	8 – 9	11
C	6, 11	4 – 5 mo	6 – 7	11 – 12	13 – 15
P1	5, 12	1½ – 1¾ yr	5 – 6	10 – 11	12 – 13
P2	4, 13	2 – 2¼ yr	6 – 7	10 – 12	12 – 14
M1	3, 14	At birth	2½ – 3	6 – 7	9 – 10
M2	2, 15	2½ – 3 yr	7 – 8	12 – 13	14 – 16
M3	1, 16	7 – 9 yr	12 – 16	17 – 21	18 – 25

Maxillary teeth

Right 1   2   3   4   5   6   7   8 | 9 10 11 12 13 14 15 16 Left
       32 31 30 29 28 27 26 25 | 24 23 22 21 20 19 18 17

Mandibular teeth

Continue

Tooth		First evidence of calcification	Crown completed (years)	Emergence (Eruption)(years)	Root completed (years)
I1	24, 25	3 – 4 mo	4 – 5	6 – 7	9
I2	23, 26	3 – 4 mo	4 – 5	7 – 8	10
C	22, 27	4 – 5 mo	6 – 7	9 – 10	12 – 14
P1	21, 28	1¼– 2 yr	5 – 6	10 – 12	12 – 13
P2	20, 29	2¼– 2½ yr	6 – 7	11 – 12	13 – 14
M1	19, 30	At birth	2½– 3	6 – 7	9 – 10
M2	18, 31	2½– 3 yr	7 – 8	11 – 13	14 – 15
M3	17, 32	8 – 10 yr	12 – 16	17 – 21	18 – 25

I1, central incisor; I2, lateral incisor; C, canine; P1, first premolar; P2, second premolar; M1, first molar; M2, second molar; M3, third molar.

The maxillary canines occasionally erupt along with the second molars, but in most instances of normal eruption, the canines precede them somewhat.

The **third molars** do not come in until the age 17 or later. Considerable posterior jaw growth is required after the age of 12 to allow room for these teeth (Figure 1-24). Third molars are subject to many anomalies and variations of form. Insufficient jaw development for their accommodation complicates matters in the majority of cases. Individuals who have properly developed third molars in good alignment are very much in the minority. Third-molar anomalies and variations with the complications brought about by misalignment and subnormal jaw

development comprise a subject too vast to be covered here. Figure 1-25 shows an anatomical specimen with a full complement of 32 teeth.

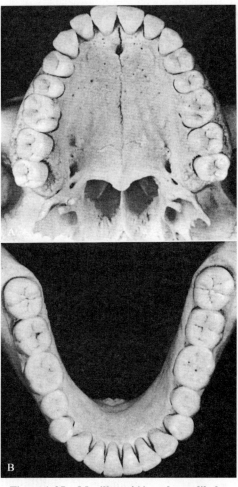

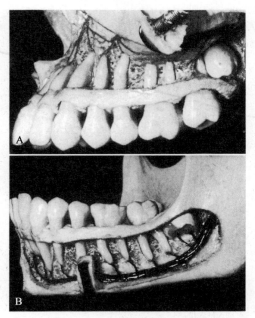

Figure 1-24   Development of the maxillary and mandibular third molars

Figure 1-25   Maxillary (A) and mandibular (B) arches with full complement of 32 teeth

Size of teeth

The size of teeth is largely genetically determined. However, marked racial differences do exist, as with the Lapps, a population with perhaps the smallest teeth, and the Australian aborigines, with perhaps the largest teeth. Gender-size dimorphism differences average about 4% and are the greatest for the maxillary canine and the least for the incisors. Often encountered is disharmony between the size of the teeth and bone size.

1. 1. 7. 9   Dental pulp

The **dental pulp** is a connective tissue organ containing a number of structures, among which are arteries, veins, a lymphatic system, and nerves. Its primary function is to form the dentin of the tooth. When the tooth is newly erupted, the dental pulp is large; it becomes progressively smaller as the tooth is completed. The pulp is relatively large in primary teeth and also in young permanent teeth. The teeth of children and young people are more sensitive than the teeth of older people to thermal change and dental operative procedures (heat generation). The opening of the pulp cavity at the apex is constricted and is called the **apical foramen.** The pulp keeps its tissue-forming function (e. g. to form **secondary dentin**), especially with the advance of dental caries toward the pulp. The pulp cavity becomes smaller and more constricted with age. The pulp chamber within the crown may become almost obliterated with a secondary deposit. This process is not so extensive in deciduous teeth.

1. 1. 7. 10   Cementoenamel junction

At the cementoenamel junction (CEJ) (see Figures 1-3 and 1-4), visualized anatomically as the cervical line, the following several types of junctions are found: ① the enamel overlapping the cementum, ② an end-to-end approximating junction, ③ the absence of connecting enamel and cementum so that the dentin is an external part of the surface of the root, and ④ an overlapping of the enamel by the cementum. These different junctions have clinical significance in the presence of disease (e. g. gingivitis, recession of the gingiva with exposure of the CEJ, loss of attachment of the supporting periodontal fibers in periodontitis); cervical sensitivity, caries, and erosion; and placement of the margins of dental restorations.

The CEJ is a significant landmark for probing the level of the attachment of fibers to the tooth in the presence of periodontal diseases. Using a periodontal probe (Figure 1-26 A), it is possible to relate the position of the gingival margin and the attachment to the CEJ (see Figure 1-26 B). Probing is done clinically to determine the level of periodontal support [i. e. regardless of whether a loss of periodontal attachment due to periodontal disease has occurred, as with pathologically deepened gingival crevices (periodontal pockets)]. The clinician should be able to envision the CEJ of each tooth and relate it to areas of risk. The enamel extension is apical to its normal CEJ level and is a risk factor for periodontal disease because the periodontal fibers, which are imbedded in cementum to support the tooth, are not in their usual position and do not act as a barrier to the advance of periodontal disease. In effect, the **epithelial attachment** over the surface of the enamel, which does not have this kind of attachment, may become detached in the narrow and difficult-to-clean bifurcation area because of plaque and calculus. Thus enamel projections into buccal and lingual bifurcations are considered to increase vulnerability to the advance of periodontal disease.

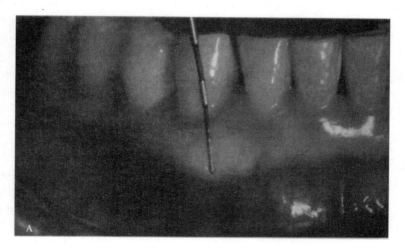

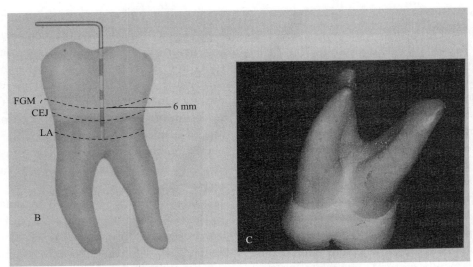

Figure 1-26 A. Periodontal probe divided into 3-mm segments. **B.** Probe at the level of attachment (LA). Probe indicates a pathologically deepened crevice of 6mm and a loss of attachment of 3+ mm. **C.** Enamel projection into the bifurcation of a mandibular molar. CEJ, cementoenamel junction; FGM, free gingival margin
(A from Perry DA, Beemsterboer PL. Periodontology for the dental hygienist. 3rd ed. St. Louis: Saunders, 2007.)

Thus the **location** and **nature** of the CEJ are more than descriptive terms used simply to describe some aspect of tooth morphology; they have some clinical significance. This consideration is also true for the cervical line; it is more than just a line of demarcation between the anatomical crown and the root of a tooth. It may be necessary to determine the nature, location, and pathological changes occurring at the CEJ to make a diagnosis of and to treat, for example, cervical caries, keeping in mind that the CEJ generally lies apical to the epithelial attachment and gingival margin in young adults.

1.1.8   Dental Age

Dental age is generally based on the formation or eruption of the teeth. The latter is usually based on the time that the teeth emerge through the mucous membrane or gingiva, which is, in effect, a single event for each tooth. However, the formation of teeth can be viewed as being continuous throughout the juvenile years. When the last tooth has been completed, the skeleton is approaching complete maturation. Later attrition and wear may be used to estimate chronological age, but the estimation of adult age at best is only on the order of ±5 years. Estimation of juvenile age is more precise than that of adult age.

Chronologies of prenatal tooth formation are based generally on dissected fetal material (see Figures 1-13 and 1-17); postnatal development chronol-

ogies are most often based on radiological data (Figures 1-27 and 1-28), but not always. Thus chronologies based on any single method are not usually feasible.

The dentition may be considered to be the single best physiological indicator of chronological age in juveniles. The knowledge of dental age has practical clinical applications; however, it is recognized that the coverage of these applications here must be brief. When indicated, references to a more detailed coverage are provided. Values for predicting age from stages of the formation of permanent mandibular teeth are considered in the section tooth formation standards in this chapter.

Dental age has been assessed on the basis of the basis of the number of the teeth at each chronological age or on stages of the formation of crowns and roots of the teeth. Dental age during the mixed dentition period (transition from primary to permanent dentition) may be assessed on the basis of which teeth have erupted, the amount of resorption of the roots of primary teeth, and the amount of development of the permanent teeth.

Dental age can reflect an assessment of physiological age comparable to age based on skeletal development, weight, or height. When the teeth are forming, the crowns and roots of the teeth appear to be the tissues least affected by environmental influences (nutrition, endocrinopathies, etc.); however, when a substance such as the antibiotic tetracycline (Figure 1-29 A) is ingested by the mother during

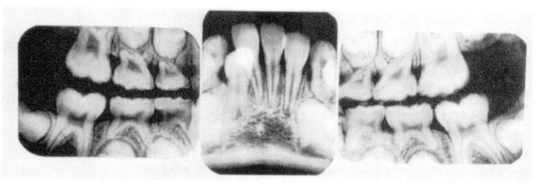

Figure 1-27   Shown in this radiograph are 6-year molars in position, roots of primary teeth being resorbed, and formation of succedaneous teeth

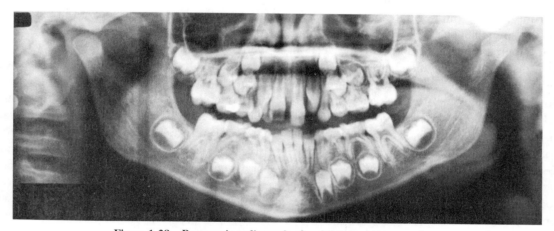

Figure 1-28   Panoramic radiograph of a child about 7 years of age
This type of examination is of great value in registering an overall record of development
(From Pappas GC, Wallace WR. Panoramic sialography. Dent Radiogr Photogr, 1970, 43:27.)

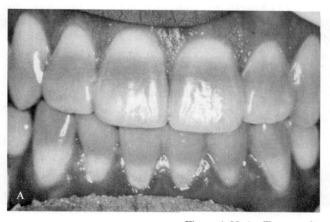 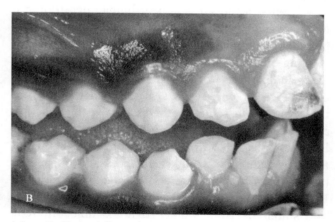

Figure 1-29 A. Tetra cycline staining. **B.** Enamel fluorosis
(From Neville BW, Damm DD, Allen CM, et al. Oral and maxillofacial pathology. 3rd ed. St. Louis: Saunders, 2009.)

certain times of the development of the dentitions, significant discoloration from yellow to brown to bluish violet from part (cervical) to all of the enamel may occur.

The benefits of fluoride for the control of dental caries are well established. However, its widespread use has resulted in an increasing prevalence of fluorosis (Figure 1-29 B) in both nonfluoridated and optimally fluoridated populations. Parents should be advised about the best early use of fluoride to reduce the prevalence of clinically noticeable fluorosis. Children under age 6 should use only a pea-sized amount of fluoride toothpaste; parents should consult their dentists concerning the use of fluoride toothpaste by children under age 2 years.

Dental development may be based also on the emergence (eruption) of the teeth; however, because caries, tooth loss, and severe malnutrition may influence the emergence of teeth through the gingiva, chronologies of the eruption of teeth are less satisfactory for dental age assessment than those based on tooth formation. In addition, tooth formation may be divided appropriately into a number of stages that cover continuously the development of teeth in contrast to the single episode of tooth eruption. The stages of development are considered in the section tooth formation standards in this chapter.

The importance of the emergence of the teeth to the development of oral motor behavior is often overlooked, undoubtedly partly as a result of the paucity of information available. However, the appearance of the teeth in the mouth at a strategic time in the maturation of the infant's nervous system and its interface with the external environment must have a profound effect on the neurobehavioral mechanisms underlying the infant's development and learning of feeding behavior, particularly the acquisition of masticatory skills.

1.1.8.1   Tooth formation standards

Events in the formation of human dentition are based primarily on data from studies of dissected prenatal anatomic material and from radiographic imaging of the teeth of the same subjects over time (longitudinal data) or of different subjects of different ages seen once (cross-sectional data). From these kinds of studies both descriptive information and chronological data may be obtained. To assemble a complete description or chronology of human tooth formation, it would seem necessary to use data based on more than one source and methodology. However, it is not easy to define ideal tooth formation standards from studies that examine different variables and use many different statistical methods. Subjects surveyed in most studies of dental development are essentially of European derivation, and population differences can only be established by studies that share methodology and information on tooth formation in populations of nonwhite/non-European ancestry.

The age of emergency of teeth has been established for a number of population groups, but much less is known about chronologies of tooth formation.

(Haiou Jia　贾海欧)

1.2   Structures of the Oral Cavity

1.2.1   The Oral Cavity

The term **oral cavity** is used when referring to the inner portion of the mouth. The oral cavity extends from the anterior opening at the lips to the oro-pharynx, or throat posteriorly. The palate, or roof of the mouth, is the superior, or upper, border; and the tongue, along with the musculature beneath it, defines the inferior or lower boundary.

The soft, moist tissue called the **mucous membrane** lines the oral cavity. In the mouth, the mucous membrane is referred to as the **oral mucosa**. The oral mucosa is pink and occurs in various degrees of thickness. Although not as strong or as thick as skin, it acts as a protective covering for the oral cavity. In some areas the oral mucosa is firmly attached, as on the gingiva and hard palate. In other areas, such as the cheek, it is much looser. There are three types of oral mucosa, each classified according to function and location:

(1) **Masticatory mucosa** covers areas subject to stress, such as gingival tissue and the hard palate.

(2) **Specialized mucosa** covers the area that has the specific function of taste on the dorsum of the tongue.

(3) **Lining mucosa** covers all other areas of the oral cavity, such as the inner surfaces of the lips and cheeks and the floor and roof of the mouth.

1.2.2   Divisions

The oral cavity is divided into two sections, the oral vestibule and the oral cavity proper. The oral vestibule is the area between the inner lips, or labial mucosa, and cheeks (buccal mucosa) and the front (facial) surfaces of the teeth. The **oral cavity proper** extends from the inner (lingual) surfaces of the teeth to the oro-pharynx.

1.2.3   Functions

Chewing of food, or mastication, is the most obvious function of the oral cavity. As chewing occurs, food is moistened with saliva, preparing it for swallowing (deglutition) and digestion. The tongue is the taste organ for food and assists the cheek and lip muscles with movement of food around the oral cavity. In addition to these functions, the oral cavity provides an air passage and assists the tongue with speech.

1.2.4　Structures External to the Oral Cavity

The structures of the lips, cheeks, and related areas of the face are closely associated with the oral cavity because they assist with its effective functioning. These outer structures are made up of muscles that aid in opening and closing the lips, and compressing food against as well as moving it away from the teeth. They include:

Labial commissure: the closure line of the lips.

Philtrum: shallow depression extending from the area below the middle of the nose to the center of the upper lip.

Vermilion zone: the pink border of the lips (thinly keratinized epithelium).

Naso-labial groove: a shallow depression extending from the corner of the nose (ala) to the corner of the lips.

Labio-mental groove: a shallow linear depression between the center of the lower lip and the chin.

Labial tubercle: a small projection in the middle of the upper lip that may enlarge or thicken.

1.2.5　Structures of the Oral Vestibule

Although the oral vestibule is a small antechamber, it contains several structures that should be recognized (Figure 1-30).

Labial frenum: an elevated fold of soft mucous tissue extending from the alveolar mucosa of the two central incisors to the labial mucosa (A superior frenum exists in the maxillary area, an inferior frenum is located in the mandibular area).

Buccal frenum: an elevated fold of soft tissue extending from the alveolar mucosa above the canine or premolar to the buccal mucosa.

Maxillary tuberosity: a small, rounded extension of bone, covered with soft tissue, posterior to the last maxillary tooth.

Retromolar area: a triangular area of bone, covered with soft tissue, posterior to the last mandibular tooth.

Stensen's papilla: a small, raised flap of soft tissue on the buccal mucosa opposite the maxillary molar (It is often marked with a tiny red dot, which is the opening to the parotid or Stensen's salivary gland).

Linea alba: a raised, white horizontal extension of soft tissue along the buccal mucosa at the occlusal line (The literal translation of these words is "white line". The linea alba is not present in all mouths).

Gingiva: pink, stippled mucosa surrounding the necks of the teeth and covering the bone in which the teeth are anchored.

Fordyce granules: small, yellow spots on the buccal mucosa and inner lip. They are sebaceous glands and have no clinical significance.

Anterior tonsillar pillar: folds of tissue that extend horizontally from the uvula to the base of the tongue.

Posterior tonsillar: a set of arches of tissue set farther back in the throat than the anterior tonsillar pillar.

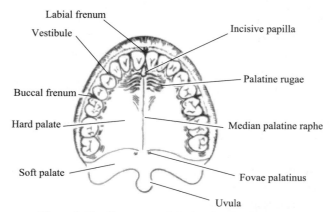

Figure 1-30　Structures of the hard and soft palates

1.2.6　Structures of the Oral Cavity Proper

1. 2. 6. 1　Roof of the mouth

When the mouth is wild open, it is possible to observe all the structures of the oral cavity proper. The following structures are located on the roof of the mouth (see Figure 1-30):

Palate: the concave surface that is known as the roof of the mouth and is divided into the hard and soft palate.

Hard palate: the bony anterior two-thirds of the palate that is covered with mucosa.

Soft palate: the posterior third of the palate, made up of muscular fibers covered with mucosa (It is a deeper color pink than the hard palate because of its highly vascular composition).

Palatine torus: a bony prominence of varied size located at the midline of the hard palate (It is a non-pathologic excess of bone covered with mucosa and only is present in about 20 percent of the population).

Incisive papilla: a small, raised, rounded structure of soft tissue at the anterior midline of the hard palate (It is directly behind the two maxillary central incisors and covers and protects the incisive foramen, an opening in the bone directly beneath it through which nerves and blood vessels travel).

Palatine raphe: a junction of soft tissue extending vertically along the entire middle of the hard palate. Also known as the median palatine raphe.

Palatine rugae: paired raised, palatine folds of soft tissue on the anterior portion of the hard palate. The rugae extend horizontally from the raphe and prevent food from adhering to the palate.

Fovea palatinus: two small indentations, one on either side of the raphe, located at the junction of the hard and soft palate (These are remnants of minor salivary glands. Their only value is as the terminal demarcation in the fabrication of the maxillary denture).

Uvula: a downward projection of the soft palate made up of connective tissue, muscles, and glands.

1.2.6.2   Fauces

The following structures are located at the posterior portion of the oral cavity and from the pillars of fauces, the arch or entryway that joins the oral cavity with the pharynx.

Oro-pharynx: the area of the oral cavity that joins it with the throat or pharynx (On either side are the arches of muscular tissue called the pillars of fauces).

Glossopharyngeal muscle: the anterior pillar of fauces extending from the outer surface of the palate to the tongue.

Palatopharyngeal muscle: the posterior pillar of fauces extending from the pharynx to the palate.

Palatine tonsils: masses of lymphoid tissue located between the anterior and posterior pillars of fauces.

1.2.6.3   Tongue

The tongue is a muscular structure covered with oral mucosa. The anterior two-thirds of the tongue is referred to as the body; the posterior third is the base of the tongue. The following structures are located on the **dorsum** of the tongue, as shown in Figure 1-31.

Median sulcus: a shallow groove extending along the midline of the tongue, ending in a slight depression called the foramen caecum.

Foramen caecum: a "V" shaped terminal sulcus at the posterior area of the median sulcus. It is considered the junction of the oral and pharyngeal sections of the tongue.

There are numerous **papillae** on the dorsum of the tongue:

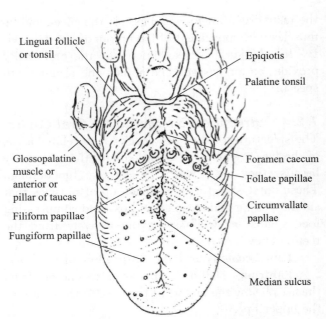

Figure 1-31   Structures on the tongue

Circumvallate from a "V" shape and are anterior to the foramen caecum. They vary from 8 to 10 in number and are the largest of the papillae.

Fungiform are located on the sides and apex of the tongue, although they can appear on other portions as well. These are broad, round, red toadstool-shaped papillae.

Filiform are abundantly located on the anterior two-thirds of the tongue. These long, thin, more flexible papillae are greyish in color.

Foliate are located on the lateral surfaces of the posterior third of the tongue. There are 3 − 5 (or more) of these large raised papillae on each side.

The tongue functions as the main organ of taste and is an important adjunct of speech. It also assists in mastication by rolling and kneading the food against the teeth and hard palate, and in deglutition by pushing the food backward into the oro-pharynx.

Taste buds are located in the papillae of the tongue and are stimulated when food is dissolved. The four primary taste sensations are bitter, sweet, salty, and sour (acid) (Table 1-3).

Table 1-3   The primary tastes that stimulate the papillae

Papillae	Taste
Circumvallate	Bitter
Fungiform	Sweet, sour, salty
Foliate	Sour
Filiform	Rarely have taste buds

The base of the tongue is attached. It is continuous with the oral portion, extending downward toward the epiglottis. The lingual tonsils (or lingual follicles), located on the sides of the posterior median line, are nodular masses of lymphoid follicles.

The following structures are located on the floor of the oral cavity. In order for these structures to be observed, the tongue must be raised, as shown in Figure 1-32.

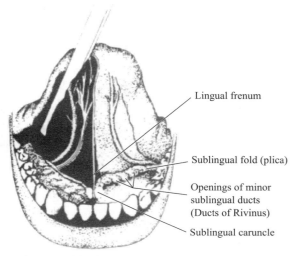

Lingual frenum

Sublingual fold (plica)

Openings of minor sublingual ducts (Ducts of Rivinus)

Sublingual caruncle

Figure 1-32　Structures on the floor of the mouth

Lingual frenum: an elevated fold of soft tissue located on the floor of the mouth at the midline. It extends from the tissue below the central incisors to the undersurface of the tongue.

Sublingual caruncles: round, elevated sections of soft tissue on either side of the lingual frenum, directly behind the central incisors on the floor of the mouth. Within the caruncles are duct openings to the sublingual (Bartholin's) and submandibular (Wharton's) salivary glands.

Sublingual fold: an elevated fold of soft tissue extending, medial, along the floor of the mouth toward the tongue. This fold contains the opening to salivary glands called the **Ducts of Rivinus.**

Mandibular tori: an overgrowth of bone occurring bilaterally on the internal borders of the mandible. As with the maxillary torus, this overgrowth is nonpathologic and occurs in only 8 percent of the population.

■ Summary

Dental anatomy is about the development, morphology, function, and identity of each of the teeth in the human dentitions, as well as the way in which the teeth relate in shape, form, structure, color, and function to the other teeth in the same dental arch and to the teeth in the opposing arch.

The structures external to the oral cavity include the lips, cheeks, and related areas of the face that assist the oral cavity in functioning effectively.

The entire oral cavity, or mouth, is lined with a soft, moist covering called the oral mucosa. This lining has different degrees of consistency that enhance and protect oral structures such as the tongue and hard palate.

The oral cavity is divided into two sections: the oral vestibule and the oral cavity proper, each with its associated structures. It is important to be familiar with the complete anatomy of the oral structures as well as with the terminology necessary for differentiating normal from abnormal.

■ Questions

1. How many deciduous teeth are there in the mouth?
2. How many permanent teeth are there in the mouth?
3. The border of the oral cavity?
4. The function of the oral cavity?

(Rudong Xing　邢汝东)

References

[1] Garn SM. Variability of tooth formation. J Dent Res, 1959, 38 (1): 135-148.

[2] Alvarez J, Navia JM. Nutritional status, tooth eruption and dental caries: a review. Am J Clin Nutr, 1989, 49 (3): 417-426.

[3] Ronnerman A. The effect of early loss of primary molars on tooth eruption and space conditions: a longitudinal study. Acta Odontol Scand, 1977, 35 (5): 229-239.

[4] Garn SM, Lewis AB, Kerewsky RS, et al. Genetic, nutri-

tional, and maturational correlates of dental development. J Dent Res, 1965, 44: 228-242.

[5] Falkner F. Deciduous tooth eruption. Arch Dis Child, 1957,32 (165): 386-391.

[6] Lunt RC, Law DB. A review of the chronology of deciduous teeth. J Am Dent Assoc, 1974, 89 (3): 599-606.

[7] Garn SM, Lewis AB, Kerewsky RS. Relationship between sexual dimorphism in tooth size as studied within families. Arch Oral Biol, 1967, 12 (2): 299-301.

[8] Hojo M. On the pattern of the dental abrasion. Okajimas Folia Anat Jpn, 1954, 26 (1-2): 11-30.

[9] Moorrees CF, Fanning EA, Hunt EE Jr, et al. Age variation of formation stages for ten permanent teeth. J Dent Res, 1963, 42: 1490-1502.

[10] Anderson DL, Thompson GW, Popovich F. Age of attainment of mineralization stages of the permanent dentition. J Forensic Sci, 1976, 21 (1): 191-200.

[11] Garn SM, Lewis AB, Polacheck DL. Variability of tooth formation in man. Science, 1958, 128 (3337): 1510.

[12] Demirjian A, Levesque GY. Sexual differences in dental development and prediction of emergence. J Dent Res, 1980, 59 (7): 1110-1122.

[13] Demisch A, Wartman P. Calcification of the mandibular third molar and its relation to skeletal and chronological age in children. Child Dev, 1956, 27 (4): 459-473.

[14] Haataia J. Development of the mandibular permanent teeth of Helsinki children. Suom Hammaslaak Toim, 1965, 61: 43-53.

[15] Fass EN. A chronology of growth of the human dentition. ASDC J Dent Child, 1969, 36 (6): 391-401.

[16] Wolanski N. A new method for the evaluation of tooth formation. Acta Genet Stat Med, 1966, 16 (2): 186-197.

[17] Nyström M, Haataja J, Kataja M, et al. Dental maturity in Finnish children, estimated from the development of seven permanent mandibular teeth. Acta Odontol Scand, 1986, 44 (4): 193-198.

[18] Sato S, Ogiwara Y. Biostatistic study of the eruption order of deciduous teeth. Bull Tokyo Dent Coll, 1971, 12 (1): 45-76.

[19] Marjorie J Short. Head, Neck & Dental Anatomy. 3rd ed. Canada: Thomson Delmar Learning, 2002.

[20] Pi Xin. Oral Anatomy and Physiology. 5th ed. Beijing: People' Medical Publishing House,2003.

Chapter 2

Cariology and Endodontics

▪ Objectives

To explain the etiology, clinical presentation and treatment of tooth hard tissue diseases and diseases of pulp and periapical tissues, with emphasis on dental caries, pulpitis and periodontitis.

▪ Key Concepts

Clinical presentation of dental caries, etiology of dental caries, fundamental principles and procedures of cavity preparation, bacterial cause in pulpitis and periodontitis, clinical presentation of acute and chronic pulpitis, as well as acute and chronic apical periodontitis, procedure of root canal therapy.

▪ Introduction

Dental caries is one of the most common chronic diseases in the world. It is ubiquitous in all populations throughout the world and is the key factor responsible for dental pain and tooth loss. It can ultimately result in demineralization of the mineral portion of tooth hard tissue followed by disintegration of the organic material. Progression of the lesion into dentine can eventually lead to bacterial invasion and necrosis of the pulp and spread of infection into the periapical tissues, thus causing pain and even tooth loss.

Direct injury of the pulp from caries occurs via the dentinal tubules. As a consequence of pathologic changes in the dental pulp, the root canal system can harbor numerous irritants. Depending on the nature and quantity of these irritants, as well as the duration of exposure of the periradicular tissues, a variety of tissue inflammatory changes can occur because irritants from the infected root canal system through tubules, lateral or accessory canals, furcation canals, and the apical foramina may directly affect the surrounding attachment apparatus. Varied clinical symptoms ranging from extremely intolerable pain to vague discomfort coincide accordingly.

This chapter of "cariology and endodontics" focuses on the aforementioned most important and most commonly encountered dental diseases: dental caries and diseases in pulp and periapical tissues, with emphasis on etiology, clinical presentation and treatment.

2.1 Dental Caries

Dental caries, or tooth decay, is an infectious microbiological disease that results in localized dissolution and destruction of the calcified tissues of the teeth.

Dental caries is one of the most common chronic diseases in the world. It is ubiquitous in all populations throughout the world and is the key factor responsible for dental pain and tooth loss. The carious process affects the mineralized tissues of the teeth, namely enamel, dentine, and cementum, and is caused by the action of microorganisms on fermentable carbohydrates in the diet. It can ultimately result in demineralization of the mineral portion of these tissues followed by disintegration of the organic material. Progression of the lesion into dentine can eventually lead to bacterial invasion and necrosis of the pulp and spread of infection into the periapical tissues, thus causing pain and even tooth loss.

The first sign of a caries lesion on enamel that can be detected with the naked eye is often called a white-spot lesion. In other words, an initial lesion appears as a white, opaque change (a white spot). Dental caries is a chronic disease, a process that progresses very slowly in most individuals. The disease is seldom self-limiting and, in the absence of treatment, caries progresses into destruction of the tooth and eventual infection of the dental pulp.

2.1.1 Etiology

The factors involved in the caries process, which include dental plaque, diet, host and teeth, as well as time were presented in the 1960s in a model of overlapping circles.

Dental plaque

The prevalence of mutans streptococci and lactobacilli is associated with dental caries. *Streptococcus mutans* is involved in caries formation from its initiation, while lactobacilli are so-called secondary organisms that flourish in a carious environment and contribute to caries progression. *Streptococcus mutans* and lactobacilli can produce great amounts of acids (acidogenic); are tolerant of acidic environ-

ments (aciduric); are vigorously stimulated by sucrose.

Diet

Dietary carbohydrates are necessary for the bacteria to produce the acids that initiate demineralization.

Host and teeth

Flow rate and buffering capacity may be the most important protective qualities of saliva. Both help neutralize and clear the acids and carbohydrates from dental plaque.

Time

Time indicates that the substrate (dietary sugars) must be present for a sufficient length of time to cause demineralization. On the other hand, it is clear that caries lesions do not develop overnight; in fact, it may take years for cavitation to occur.

2.1.2 Clinical Presentation

2.1.2.1 Classification of dental caries

(1) Classification according to speed of progress

An acute caries lesion is softened area that shows a yellowish or light brown discoloration. Rampant caries is the name given to multiple active carious lesions occurring in the same patient. This frequently involves surfaces of teeth that do not usually experience dental caries. Patients with rampant caries can be classified according to the assumed causality, e. g. bottle or nursing caries, baby caries, early childhood caries, radiation caries or drug-induced caries.

Some slowly progressing lesions may be brownish or back and reveal a leathery consistency on probing with moderate pressure, which are referred to as chronic caries. A lesion that may have formed years previously and then stopped further progression is referred to as an arrested caries lesion. It is considered that the lesion arrests mainly due to the altered environmental conditions owing to better use of the fully erupted teeth, which promoted natural removal of bacterial accumulations and hence lesion arrest. Most often the arrested approximal lesion is seen on teeth where the adjacent tooth has been extracted, where the local environmental conditions have been changed completely.

Cries lesions develop adjacent to a filling are commonly referred to as secondary caries.

(2) Classification according to anatomical site

Lesions may commonly be found in pits and fissures or on smooth surfaces. Smooth-surface lesions may start on enamel (enamel caries) or on the exposed root cementum and dentin (root caries).

Numerous epidemiological data and common clinical experience have repeatedly shown that occlusal surfaces of posterior teeth are the most vulnerable sites for dental caries. Conventionally, the high incidence of caries on these surfaces has been directly related to the narrow and inaccessible pits and fissures on occlusal surfaces. Because enamel demineralization always follows the rods, it is natural that the enamel lesion initiated in a fossa gradually assumes the shape of a cone with its base towards the enamel-dentinal junction. In a fossa where several surfaces are involved, the lesion entity is, in reality, shaped as a cone in three dimensions. It is called 'undermining' character of occlusal caries and this explains why the openings of occlusal cavities are always smaller than the base.

Recession of the gingival margin is inevitable result of poor oral hygiene and loss of periodontal attachment with age. As the gingival margin recedes the enamel-cementum junction becomes exposed. This region of the tooth is highly irregular and represents a particular bacterial retention site. This condition is common within the elderly population.

(3) Classification according to depth of the lesion

1) Caries in enamel: The earliest macroscopic evidence of enamel caries is known as the "white spot lesion". It is best seen on dried clean teeth surfaces where the lesion appears as a small, opaque, white area. The color of the lesion distinguishes it from the adjacent translucent sound enamel. At this stage mineral loss cannot be detected with a probe because the enamel is hard and no cavity is present. Sometimes this lesion may appear brown in color due to exogenous material absorbed into its porosities. If the lesion progresses, the surface zone eventually breaks down and a cavity forms. Plaque now forms within the cavity and may be protected from cleaning aids such as a tooth-brush filament or dental flows. For this reason a cavitated lesion is more likely to progress.

Diagnosis of smooth surface enamel caries can be gained with sharp eyes at the stage of the white or brown spot lesion before cavitation has occurred, provided the teeth are clean, dry, and well lit. Root surface caries, in its early stages, appears as one or smaller, well defined, discolored areas located in an area of plaque stagnation close to the gingival margin. Lesions may vary in color from yellowish or light brown, through midbrown to almost black. Root surface lesions tend to spread laterally and coalesce with minor neighboring lesions and may thus eventually encircle the tooth.

While caries on free smooth surfaces is easy to see, caries in pits and fissures is difficult to diagnose at this early stage. It is suggested that sharp eyes be used to pick up discoloration and cavitation. Bitewing radiographs are of great importance in the detection of occlusal caries, although by the time a lesion can be seen radiographically it is well into dentine.

2) Caries in dentine: It has been stated that enamel carious lesions on smooth surfaces and in fissures differ in shape because of the anatomy of the fissure and the direction of the enamel prisms. The smooth surface lesion is cone shaped, the base of the cone being at the enamel surface. The fissure lesion is also ultimately cone shaped but the base of the cone is at the enamel-dentine junction. This is because the spread of the enamel lesion is guided by prism direction and hence the fissure lesion broadens as it approaches the dentine.

When and if the carious process reaches the enamel-dentine junction, caries appears to spread laterally along the junction to involve the dentine on a wider front. Sound enamel appears to be undermined by the carious process in dentine and the resulting lesion is larger than would be expected from examination of the enamel alone, particularly in fissure lesions. The apparent undermining of enamel by the carious process is of relevance in cavity preparation because enamel must often be removed to gain access to the soft and infected carious dentine beneath it.

The dentin and the pulp are classically described as two separate tissues, although the dentin is merely the product of the differentiated pulpal odontoblasts. Therefore the pulp and the dentin should be regarded as a single unit. Dentin is a vital, highly mineralized tissue capable of responding to stimuli as long as the pulp remains alive. Thus, pain may be one of the immediate responses to stimulation of odontoblasts, and this can occur when irritants such as acid in caries reach the dentinoenamel junction (or the ends of the odontoblastic processes).

The purpose of a bitewing radiograph is to detect lesions that are clinically hidden from a careful clinical visual examination. It is a useful technique where an adjacent tooth prevents the dentist from seeing an approximal lesion. The radiograph will also help to estimate the depth of the lesion, although lesions apparently confined to the inner enamel on radiography are in dentin histologically. Bitewing radiographs should always be examined for occlusal caries in dentin.

2.2 Treatment for Dental Caries

2.2.1 Fissure Sealants
There is ample evidence that caries does not progress as long as the fissure remains sealed. Thus, sealing appears very effective in conserving sound tooth structure. An unfilled or lightly filled resin is used to penetrate the fissures and prevent plaque accumulation on the occlusal surface. A fissure sealant has the advantage that the tooth does not have to be cut and no irreversible intervention is involved. Active lesions covered by the resin do not progress further and the possible development of new lesions at other sites in the fissure is prevented.

Treatment procedures include cleaning, isolation, etching, sealant application and light curing.

2.2.2 Operative Management of Dental Caries
2.2.2.1 Cavity preparation

This involves accessing the demineralized soft dentin, removing most of the infected dental tissue and adjusting the remaining cavity so that the filling material of choice can be applied.
Classification for cavities

As early as 1908, GV Black published a classification for the preparation related to its position on the tooth. The classification is:

Class 1: lesions beginning in pits and fissures in any part of the teeth in which these occur

Class 2: lesions beginning in the proximal surfaces of the bicuspids and molars

Class 3: lesions beginning in the proximal surfaces of the incisors and cuspids, which do not require the removal and restoration of the incisal angle

Class 4: lesions beginning in the proximal surfaces of the incisors which require the removal and restoration of the incisal angle

Class 5: lesions beginning in the gingival third- not pit or fissure cavities - of the labial, buccal or lingual surfaces of the teeth.

A second type of classification is by the number of surfaces involved. The simple cavity involves only one surface, the compound cavity involves two surfaces of the tooth, and the complex cavity involves three or more surfaces.
Cavity terminology

Clinically, cavity is mentioned along with cavity terminology. Noting that the teeth have five surfaces on the clinical crown—facial/buccal, lingual/palatal, incisal/occlusal, mesial, and distal—a cavity may be classified according to the surface or surfaces involved, such as distal or mesiolingual. In writing such classification, abbreviations such as D or ML are used.
Fundamental principles of cavity preparation

In general terms the objectives of cavity preparation are to remove all defects and give the necessary protection to the pulp, to locate the margins of the restoration as conservatively as possible, to form the cavity so that under the force of mastication the tooth or the restoration or both will not fracture and the restoration will not be displaced, and to allow for the esthetic and functional placement of a restorative material.

Resistance form may be defined as that shape and placement of the cavity walls that best enable both the restoration and the tooth to withstand occlusal forces without fracture.

Retention form is that shape or form of the cavity that best permits the restoration to resist displacement through tipping or lifting forces.

2.2.2.2 Isolation

To prevent salivary contamination of the surfaces, the material should be placed under rubber dam isolation or with the help of cotton wool rolls and a saliva ejector.

2.2.2.3 Cavity sealers and bases

Cavity sealers are materials that provide a protective coating to the walls of the prepared cavity and a barrier to leakage at the interface of the restorative material and the walls.

Materials in the category of cavity bases are used to replace missing dentin, as in bulk buildup and/or in blocking out undercuts in preparations for indirect restorations. Zinc oxide-eugenol and zinc phosphate cements as well as glass ionomers have been used as bases for a variety of restorative materials.

2.2.2.4 Insertion of the restorative materials

Currently, many restorative materials are available. Clinicians have to be cognizant that the restoration should seal the cavity and not allow leakage of bacteria between the filling and the tooth. Thus the cavity sealing ability of restorative materials is important. In addition, operative dentistry should be carried out to a high standard so that restorations and the adjacent tooth surface may be kept plaque free.

2.3   Tetracycline Stained Teeth

2.3.1   Etiology and Clinical Presentation

Tetracycline is a group of broad-spectrum antibiotics that has an affinity for calcified tissue. It can cross the placental barrier to affect the deciduous teeth. If the drug is taken by infants and young children the developing permanent teeth will usually be discolored.

Tooth shades can be yellow, yellow-brown, brown, dark gray, or blue, depending on the type of tetracycline, dosage, duration of intake, and patient's age at the time of administration. Discoloration is usually bilateral, affecting multiple teeth in both arches. Deposition of the tetracycline may be continuous or laid down in stripes depending on whether the ingestion was continuous or interrupted. Repeated exposure of tetracycline-discolored tooth to ultraviolet radiation can lead to formation of a reddish-purple oxidation by-product that permanently discolors the teeth.

If tetracycline staining is to be avoided, this group of drugs should not be administered in pregnancy or to children under 12 years.

2.3.2   Treatment

Because many of these conditions do not progress, the treatment can often be deferred until the patient is concerned about the appearance. The aim of treatment is almost entirely cosmetic, but no less important for that. Where molar hypomineralization results in chipping of the enamel and plaque stagnation, a restoration may be needed so that the patient can clean.

Bleaching may be effective in some cases of tetracycline stain. Two approaches have been used to treat tetracycline discoloration: ① bleaching the external enamel surface, and ② intracoronal bleaching following intentional root canal therapy.

In most cases composite restorations or veneers of composite or porcelain, often with little or no tooth preparation, are the treatment of choice. Crowns may be necessary in the most severe cases.

2.4   Wedge-shaped Defect

These lesions are V-shaped notches located at the cervical area of the teeth.

These lesions are commonly caused by excessive toothbrushing. Acid is considered to be another reason for these lesions. It is easy to understand how tooth tissue softened by acid is particularly susceptible to wear. Another theory states that as teeth flex under occlusal load, stresses are transmitted to the cervical area causing cervical enamel rods to fracture and dislodge. Over time, with increased flexural movements, a V-shaped notch develops, and the tooth becomes weaker as tooth structure is lost and the tooth flexure increases.

Clinically, these lesions commonly present buccally at the cervical margin of first premolars.

Several preventive and restorative treatment measures for wedge-shaped defects have been proposed such as: a change of oral hygiene behavior, application of desensitization products, glass-ionomers and compomers, resin composites, occlusal adjustments if occlusal trauma coincides.

2.5   Dentine Hypersensitivity

Dentine hypersensitivity, or hypersensitive dentine, is probably a symptom complex, rather than a true disease.

2.5.1   Etiology

Dentinal sensitivity is often associated with gingival recession and noncarious cervical lesions. Sensitivity is caused by exposure of dentinal tubules that communicate between the pulp and the oral cavity; the degree of sensitivity is influenced by the number and size of the open tubules. The hydrodynamic theory is the most widely accepted explanation of dentinal sensitivity. Tactile, thermal, or osmotic stimuli can induce changes in fluid flow and elicit a pain response.

2.5.2   Clinical Presentation

The exciting factors of a hypersensitive pulp are usually cold food or drink or cold air. Sweet or sour substances, vegetable or fruit acid, or often just touching the surface with a fingernail, a toothbrush, an interdental stimulator, or an explorer may also trigger the symptom. Clinical manifestation is characterized by a short, sharp, shock—that is, "pain" best described as a sensation of sudden shock. The sensation is as sharp as it is sudden and must be elicited by some exciting factor. It is never spontaneous. The pain is of short duration, lasting only slightly longer than the time during which the irritating element is in contact with the tooth.

2.5.3 Treatment
Treatment or prevention of hypersensitivity is usually accomplished by the use of some method to occlude the open tubules, including oxalate solutions, stannous fluorides and potassium nitrate.

2.6 Incomplete Fracture or Split Tooth

2.6.1 Etiology
Most cases occur in teeth that have an opposing plunger cusp occluding centrically against a marginal ridge. The resulting horizontal forces may be the causal factor of cracked tooth.

2.6.2 Clinical Presentation
The tooth may be uncomfortable only occasionally during mastication, and at that time the pain may be one quick, unbearable stab. This is when the crack in the dentin suddenly spreads as the cusp separates from the remainder of the tooth. The most frequent complaint is that of a tooth painful to bite on, with an occasional mild ache. If the split has extended through the pulp, bacterial invasion occurs, and true pulpitis results.

2.6.3 Diagnosis
Many of the cases involve noncarious, unrestored teeth. Biting on an applicator stick or cotton roll may give the spreading action needed to elicit pain. The crown may also be painted with tincture of iodine, which is washed off after 2 minutes. The crack often appears as a dark line.

2.6.4 Treatment
Treatment involves immediate reduction of the occlusal contacts by selective grinding at the site of the crack or against the cusp or cusps of the occluding antagonist. If an incomplete fracture is suspected but the pulp is not involved, the crown should be prepared for a full crown, which should then be cemented temporarily with zinc oxide-eugenol cement.

If the incomplete fracture has entered the pulp and a true pulpalgia indicates that pulpitis is present, root canal therapy should be completed first, followed by full coverage to prevent a total fracture. If the fracture has extended completely through, into the periodontal ligament and pulp, the chances of saving the entire tooth are remote indeed.

2.7 Diseases of the Dental Pulp and Periapical Tissues

Direct injury of the pulp from caries occurs via the dentinal tubules. Irritants (bacterial by-products, disintegrating elements of carious dentin, or chemicals from foods) either permeate through tubules to contact and destroy odontoblasts and underlying cells or have an osmotic effect that also destroys cells by rapid, forceful fluid movement. The immune process and accompanying injury comprise another mechanism responsible for the development of pulpitis. As a consequence of pathologic changes in the dental pulp, the root canal system can harbor numerous irritants. Depending on the nature and quantity of these irritants, as well as the duration of exposure of the periradicular tissues, a variety of tissue changes can occur. It is believed that the egress of irritants from an infected root canal system through tubules, lateral or accessory canals, furcation canals, and the apical foramina may directly affect the surrounding attachment apparatus.

2.7.1 Etiology
Bacterial causes

Microorganisms cause virtually all pathoses of the pulp and the periradicular tissues. Invasion of the pulp cavity by bacteria is most often associated with dental caries. Importantly, bacteria and their by-products have been shown to have a direct effect on the dental pulp even without direct exposure. Fractured crown, nonfracture trauma, anomalous tract, e.g. dens invaginatus, retrogenic infection from periodontal pocket, hematogenic infection through vascular channels are other paths of invasion of bacteria.

Physical causes

Acute trauma and chronic occlusal trauma may cause the pulp vessels being either severed or smashed at the apical foramen, resulting in ischemic infarction, furthermore, pulp canal calcification, inflammation, or necrosis.

The heat generated by grinding procedures during cavity preparation, especially, without copious water coolant, may lead to ranging from reversible to irreparable changes. The pulp damage can be also caused by polishing restorations. The subsequent temperature increase gives rise to the same pulp damage previously discussed under cavity preparation.

Pulp changes are reported when amalgam was condensed into fresh cavities prepared with high-speed equipment.

Chemical causes

These consist of the chemical insult from the various filling materials.

Immunological causes

Immunocompetent cells, immunoglobulins (antibodies), and complement factors have been identified in inflamed pulpal tissues. Both the humoral and cellular responses occur in the pulp.

2.7.2 Reversible Pulpitis

The condition of reversible pulpitis is characterized by localized inflammation at the base of the involved tubules. This reactive inflammatory process resolves or diminishes with removal of the irritant.

2.7.2.1 Clinical presentation

Irreversible pulpitis is characterized by short and sharp sensation of pain. The pain is of short duration and disappears immediately after the irritating element (either hot or cold, sweet or sour) is removed from the tooth. It is never spontaneous. The suspected tooth or teeth usually present defects that allow passage of stimuli to the pulp, either from crown defects, retrograde path or occlusal trauma.

2.7.2.2 Diagnosis

A short and sharp sensation of pain caused by thermal irritant is frequently the main component of the patient's complaint. The pain must not be spontaneous. Intraoral examination notes suspected tooth or teeth with defects allowing passage of stimuli to the pulp. Cold test may cause immediate and short hyperreactive pulpalgia.

2.7.3 Irreversible Pulpitis

The pulp has been damaged beyond repair, and even with removal of the irritant it will not heal. The pulp will progressively degenerate, causing necrosis and reactive destruction. Extirpation of the pulp tissue is necessary in either pathologic process. Irreversible pulpitis can be classified into acute pulpitis

and chronic pulpitis according to clinical characteristics.

2.7.3.1 Acute pulpitis

Acute pulpitis is characterized by excruciating acute toothache.

Clinical presentation

The excruciating acute pain may be excited by heat and some patients report tooth aches at night. The pain may be spontaneous and diffuse.

Intraoral examination often reveals a huge interproximal cavity or a restoration impinging on the pulp chamber of the involved tooth, or deep periodontal pocket existing around the tooth. Violent pain may be excited during examination using explorer, and minute pulpal exposure may be also identified simultaneously.

A tooth involved in acute pulpitis is hypersensitive to thermal test. The effect of stimulus application produces a lingering effect in which the patient clearly feels that the pain is still present several seconds after stimulus removal. The involved tooth is hypersensitive to the electric pulp tester at incipient stage and less sensitive to the tester at advanced stage. The involved tooth is sometimes tender to vertical percussion at advanced stage.

Diagnosis

The violent symptom of toothache is self-incriminating. Intraoral examination reveals defect that allow passage of stimuli to the pulp. Pulp vitality test, thermal test and percussion can help locate a symptomatic tooth.

2.7.3.2 Chronic pulpitis

Chronic pulpitis is the most common pulpitis.

Clinical presentation and diagnosis

The toothache is not as violent as that in acute pulpitis, but appears vague or dull. The patients often withstand the mild symptom for weeks, months, or years. Thermal stimuli may cause the hurt and patients often report that the tooth is sore to bite. The involved tooth usually can be pointed out by the patient.

A large carious lesion is present, or a restoration is fractured or secondary caries exists. Sometimes, no pulp exposure can be identified after removal of the carious lesion and restoration, and scratching the residual dentine wall covering the pulp chamber with explorer reveals mild or no discomfort. This type of condition seems less sensitive to the pulp vitality test and thermal test, while usually tender to percussion.

If the deep cavity already extends into the pulp, the patient may report that tooth hurt when compressed by food packed into the cavity and pulp exposure is present after removal of the decayed tissue and restoration. At this level, it is referred to as chronic ulcerative pulpitis. Probing into the area of pulp exposure is not painful until deeper areas of the pulp are reached. The involved tooth appears sensitive to thermal test and insensitive to percussion.

Chronic hyperplastic pulpitis is another type of chronic pulpitis. The chronically inflamed young pulp, widely exposed by caries on its occlusal aspect, is the forerunner of this unique growth. The polyp rises out of the carious shell of the crown. The exposed tissue of a hyperplastic pulp is practically free of symptoms except that pain and hemorrhage may occur when it is stimulated directly during mastication.

2.7.4 Pulp Necrosis
As pulp inflammation progresses, the result is that the entire pulp is necrotic.
Clinical presentation and diagnosis
There are no true symptoms of complete pulp necrosis. Many cases of pulp necrosis are discovered because of the discoloration of the crown. The electric pulp tester is the instrument of choice for determining pulp necrosis. With complete necrosis, no response will be given at any level on the tester. No obvious periradicular change can be identified on the tooth with pulp necrosis radiographically.

2.7.5 Pulp Calcification
Basically, there are two distinct types of pulpal calcifications: formed structures commonly known as pulp stones and tiny crystalline masses generally termed diffuse calcifications.
Clinical presentation and diagnosis
Pulp stones of sufficient size are readily visible on radiographs. The chamber that appears to have a diffuse and obscure outline radiographically may represent a pulp that has formed large numbers of irregular pulp stones.

2.7.6 Acute Apical Periodontitis
Once bacteria have invaded the necrotic pulp, they release enzymes to break down the necrotic tissue for assimilation of the available nutrients; by the process of heterolysis, liquefaction (also called "wet gangrene") occurs. This activity produces an abundance of by-products, which eventually leak into periradicular tissues, causing inflammatory and immunologic reactions. Acute apical periodontitis is an inflammatory process in the periradicular tissues of teeth, accompanied by exudate formation within the lesion.
Clinical presentation
The early stage is a localized inflammation of the periodontal ligament in the apical region, which is associated with the exudation of plasma and emigration of inflammatory cells from the blood vessels into the periradicular tissues. Since there is little room for expansion of the periodontal ligament, increased interstitial tissue pressure can also cause physical pressure on the nerve endings, causing an intense, throbbing, periradicular pain. Sensitivity to percussion is the principal clinical feature.

Necrosis is an extension of the inflammatory cycle, which begins with acute apical periodontitis and continues to the abscess state if not checked. When abscess is confined at the periapex, acute form of periradicular pain can be most excruciating and sometimes lasts for days. The tooth is exquisitely painful to touch, and even contacting the tooth in closure may bring a flood of tears. The pain is most persistent, lasting 24 hours a day. The pain has been described as constant, gnawing, throbbing, and pounding. There is no overt swelling involved, just a grossly painful tooth elevated slightly in its socket.

Spread of abscess into the cancellous bone results in apical bone resorption. Since inflammation is not confined to the periodontal ligament but has spread to the bone, the patient now has an acute osteitis. These patients are in pain and may have systemic symptoms such as fever and increased white blood cell count. Because of the pressure from the accumulation of exudate within the confining tissues, the pain can be severe.

Necrosis of the acute abscess usually destroys enough tissue to permit fluid dispersement. Spread of the lesion toward a surface, erosion of cortical bone, and extension of the abscess through the periosteum and into the soft tissues is ordinarily accompanied by swelling and some relief. It is also quite painful, but the unbearable pain has gone and in its place is a full systolic throbbing pain, particularly on palpation. When the alveolar plate is "eroded" by the process and the abscess gathers into frank pus, the entire area softens and feels fluctuant to palpation. The involved tooth is also painful to movement or mastication.

Diagnosis

The patient has pain and, invariably, swelling. The degree of swelling varies from the initial, undetected swelling to gross cellulitis and massive asymmetry. The involved tooth also is extremely painful to percussion or palpation. Outside of percussion, electric pulp testing is the best method of diagnosis because the pulp of the tooth involved in acute apical abscess is invariably necrotic. Palpation of the area reveals the swelling, and the pressure increases the discomfort.

2.7.7 Chronic Apical Periodontitis

Clinical presentation and diagnosis

The clinical features of chronic apical periodontitis are unremarkable. The patient usually reports no significant pain, and tests reveal little or no pain on percussion. Palpation of superimposed tissues may cause discomfort. The associated tooth has a necrotic pulp and therefore should not respond to electrical or thermal stimuli.

When chronic apical periodontitis is associated with either a continuously or intermittently draining sinus tract, it is visually evident as a stoma on the oral mucosa or occasionally as a fistula on the skin of the face. The exudate can also drain through the gingival sulcus of the involved tooth.

Radiographic findings are usually associated with periradicular radiolucent changes. These changes range from thickening of the periodontal ligament and resorption of the lamina dura to destruction of apical bone resulting in a well-demarcated radiolucency. Radiographic findings are the diagnostic key.

Periradicular granuloma and periradicular cyst are two types of clinically similar chronic apical periodontitis. Radiographic findings have been used to attempt to differentiate these two lesions. The only accurate way to distinguish these two entitles is by histologic examination.

Radiographic examination of chronic apical abscess also shows the presence of bone loss at the apexes of the involved teeth.

The radiographic appearance of condensing osteitis is a well-circumscribed radiopaque area around one or all of the roots.

2.8 Endodontic Treatments

2.8.1 Emergency Treatment

Achievement of drainage and cleaning the pulpal space

For acute pulpitis, it is important to perform a pulpectomy at the emergency visit.

For acute apical periodontitis, establish drainage by access and instrumentation of the root canal. This includes introducing a small file (size 10 or 15) slightly beyond the apex to ensure patency of the canal. This is done to establish drainage from the periapical tissues. If pus continues to drain through the canal and cannot be dried within a reasonable period of time, the tooth may be left open and a cotton ball is used to prevent food impaction. These teeth can usually be closed about two days later, after additional cleaning and shaping.

Incision and drainage for swelling

Fluctuance, the sensation (on palpation) that there is fluid movement under the tissue, indicates that pus is present. With soft tissue infiltration of anesthetic around the periphery of the distended tissues, the management of this localized soft tissue swelling can be facilitated through incision and drainage of the area.

Elimination of irritants

Overmedicating the tooth may lead to acute onset of pain from medicaments that permeate into the periapical tissues. Complete elimination of the irritants from the root canal system is the treatment of choice. Calcium hydroxide intracanal dressings are therapeutic in emergency treatment.

Occlusal adjustment

Apical periodontitis caused by traumatic occlusion often results in pain on biting or eating. Occlusal adjustment is performed to remove the premature contact.

Antibiotics and analgesics

The systemic use of antibiotics in treating swellings caused by pulpal necrosis should be regarded as an aid to drainage. Patients with spreading infections or systemic signs of illness (i. e. elevated temperature or malaise) also require antibiotics. Generally the use of antibiotics alone (without concurrent attempts to establish drainage and clean the pulpal space) is not considered appropriate treatment.

2.8.2 *Treatments*

2.8.2.1 Pulp capping

Pulp capping is defined as "endodontic treatment designed to maintain the vitality of the endodontium".

Direct pulp capping

Direct pulp capping should be attempted only when a small mechanical exposure of an otherwise healthy pulp occur. In addition, aged pulp has increased fibrosis and a decreased blood supply and thus a decreased ability to mount an effective response to invading microorganisms.

The exposure should be covered with calcium hydroxide because of its documented ability to provide the highest percentage of success.

Indirect pulp capping

Several favorable conditions must be present before considering indirect pulp capping:

(1) The tooth has no history of spontaneous pain. Pulpal vitality has been confirmed with thermal or electric pulp testing.

(2) Pain elicited during pulp testing with a hot or cold stimulus should not linger after stimulus removal.

(3) A periapical radiograph should show no evidence of a periradicular lesion of endodontic origin.

The procedures are: after administering anesthesia, prepare the tooth with care in removing carious dentin near the pulp to prevent accidental pulp exposure. Place a calcium hydroxide liner over the remaining dentin. If additional sealing is indicated, use a glass-ionomer liner.

2.8.2.2 Pulpotomy

Pulpotomy involves removal of the entire coronal pulp to the level of the root orifices.

Indications

This treatment may be indicated for carious exposure and traumatic exposure (after 72 hours). Because of the reasonably good chance that the dressing will be placed on inflamed pulp, pulpotomy is contraindicated in mature teeth. However, benefits outweigh risks for this treatment in the immature tooth with incompletely formed apices and thin dentinal walls.

Treatment procedures

After anesthesia, cavity is prepared into the pulp using a sterile diamond bur of appropriate size with copious water coolant. All of the tissue in the pulp chamber should be removed. All pulp tissue that has not been removed by the round bur should be eliminated with a sharp spoon excavator. The tissue is carefully curetted from the pulp horns and other ramifications of the chamber. A thin layer of calcium hydroxide is carefully placed. The prepared cavity is filled with zinc oxide-eugenol or glass ionomer cement.

2.9 Root Canal Therapy (RCT)

The indications for endodontic therapy are legion. Every tooth, from central incisor to third molar, is a potential candidate for treatment. Modern dentistry incorporates endodontics as an integral part of restorative and prosthetic treatment. Most any tooth with pulpal involvement, provided that it has adequate periodontal support, can be a candidate for root canal treatment. Severely broken down teeth, and potential and actual abutment teeth, can be candidates for the tooth-saving procedures of endodontics.

2.9.1 *Treatment Procedures*

2.9.1.1 Root canal preparation

Access to the pulp chamber space

External outline form evolves from the internal anatomy of the tooth established by the pulp. That is to say, external outline form is established by mechanically projecting the internal anatomy of the pulp onto the external surface. This may be accomplished only by drilling into the open space of the pulp chamber and then working with the bur from the inside of the tooth to the outside, cutting away the dentin of the pulpal roof and walls overhanging the floor of the chamber. Furthermore, convenience form modifications enables unobstructed access to the canal orifice, i.e. instruments should be placed easily into the orifice of each canal without interference from overhanging walls and the clinician must be able to see each orifice and easily reach it with the instrument points.

Determination of working length

The apical constriction (minor apical diameter) is the apical portion of the root canal having the narrowest diameter. This position may vary but is usually 0.5 to 1.0 mm short of the center of the apical foramen. Therefore, it is generally accepted that the apical constriction is most frequently located 0.5 to 1.0 mm short of the radiographic apex.

Determination of working length can be obtained by radiographic methods, digital tactile sense, or electric apex locators.

Cleaning and debridement of the root canal

Instrumentation coupled with liberal irrigation will eliminate most of the bacterial contaminants of the canal as well as the necrotic debris and dentin. Enough of the dentin wall of the canal must be removed to eliminate the attached necrotic debris and, insofar as possible, the bacteria and debris found in the dentinal tubuli. Although instrumentation of the root canal is the primary method of canal debridement, irrigation is a critical adjunct. Irregularities in canal systems such as narrow isthmi and apical deltas prevent complete debridement by mechanical instrumentation alone. Irrigation serves as a physical flush to remove debris as well as serving as a bactericidal agent, tissue solvent, and lubricant.

The use of ultrasonic or sonic irrigation to better cleanse root canals of their filings, debris, and bacteria, all the way to the apex, has been well documented.

Techniques for preparing the root canal

Until now, step-back technique, step-down technique, balanced force concept using Flex-R files rotary instrumentation using nickel titanium instruments, etc, have been introduced to prepare the root canals.

2.9.1.2 Intracanal antisepsis

Residual microorganisms left in the root canal system following cleaning and shaping or microbial contamination of a root canal system between appointments have been a concern. If root canal treatment is not completed in a single appointment, antimicrobial agents are recommended for intracanal antisepsis to prevent the growth of microorganisms between appointments. The access opening in the tooth must also be sealed with an effective interappointment filling to prevent microbial contamination by microleakage from the oral cavity.

The current intracanal dressing of choice is calcium hydroxide. Although not characterized as an antiseptic, studies have shown calcium hydroxide to be an effective antimicrobial agent.

Laser intracanal irradiation may be used in this procedure, due to temperature rise. Several studies have evaluated the effectiveness of lasers in sterilizing root canals. In this sense, lasers are being used as a coadjuvant tool in endodontic therapy, for bacterial reduction, and to modify the root canal surface.

2.9.1.3 Root canal obturation

The preliminary objectives of operative endo-

dontics are total debridement of the pulpal space, development of a fluid-tight seal at the apical foramen, and total obliteration of the root canal.

The root canal is ready to be filled when the canal is cleaned and shaped to an optimum size and dryness. The tooth should be comfortable.

Materials used in obturation

Gutta-percha is by far the most universally used solid-core root canal filling material, which must be cemented into place to be effective.

The sealers are to form a fluid-tight seal at the apex by filling the minor interstices between the solid material and the wall of the canal, and also by filling patent accessory canals and multiple foramina. Zinc oxide-eugenol (ZOE) cement, calcium hydroxide sealers, sealer containing iodoform, sealers based resin chemistry are materials of choice.

Methods of obturating the root canal space

Lateral compaction of cold gutta-percha points with sealer has long been the standard against which other methods of canal obturation have been judged. This technique encompasses first placing a sealer lining in the canal. Followed by a measured primary point, that in turn is compacted laterally by a plugger-like tapering spreader to make room for additional accessory points. The final mass of points is severed at the canal's coronal orifice with a hot instrument, and final vertical compaction is done with a large plugger.

In vertical compaction of warm gutta-percha, the non-standardized cone-shaped gutta-percha points are used as the master cone. After insert the master cone, the heat carrier warms the coronal portion of the gutta-percha. A plugger is immediately inserted in the canal and the warmed gutta-percha is compacted vertically, and the material flows into and seals the apical portals of exit. "Backpacking" the remainder of the canal completes the obturation.

2.9.2 Microscopic Endodontics

Microsurgery is limited to a surgical procedure on exceptionally small and complex structures with the aid of an operation microscope. The surgical operating microscope provides the necessary illumination with a bright, focused light and magnification up to $32\times$. This enhanced visibility allows the surgeons to locate and treat anatomic variations that previously would have escaped their attention. These include the partial or complete isthmus, multiple foramina, C-shaped canals, and apical root fractures. These variations often cannot be treated by nonsurgical means.

■ Summary

Dental caries is a multifactorial disease with infectious microbiological initiation. Clinical presentation of dental caries is characterized by discoloration, cavitation and softened tooth hard tissue. Visual examination, examination by probe and radiograph facilitate diagnosis. Preventive measurements, e. g. fissure sealant, have been improved effective. However, operative treatment is of necessity for carious cavity and fundamental principles have to be followed during the procedure.

Pulpitis is a series of diseases originating from inflammation in the pulp tissue, which mainly caused by carious invasion through dentinal tubules. Clinically, varied symptoms, namely tooth pain, exist due to different stage of the pulpal inflammation. The key point of diagnosis is to clarify the symptomatic tooth or teeth. History, pulp test and radiograph are among the important diagnostic procedures.

Periodontitis is referred to as inflammatory pathoses of the periodontal tissue. Microbiological invasion from the infected root canal system is one of the most common causes. Acute apical periodontitis induces extreme agony and maybe systematic response, even life threatening. Emergency treatment has to be performed for this condition.

Root canal therapy is generally selected for pulpitis and periodontitis. It is composed of root canal preparation, intracanal antisepsis and root canal obturation.

■ Questions

1. Describe the clinical differences among dental caries, pulpitis and periodontitis?
2. What is the main principle in treating dental caries, pulpitis and periodontitis?

(**Xiaomei Hou** 侯晓玫)

References

[1] Harris RJ. Mechanisms of Hard Tissue Destruction. New York: Academic Press, 1963: 261-283.
[2] Carlsson J, Grahnen H, Jonsson G. Lactobacilli and streptococci in the mouth of children. Caries Res, 1975, 9(5): 333-339.
[3] Mjör A, Toffenetti F. Secondary caries: a literature review with case reports. Quintessence Int, 2000, 31(3): 165-179.
[4] Carvalho JC, Ekstrand KR, Thylstrup A. Dental plaque and caries on occlusal surfaces of first permanent molars in relation to stage of eruption. J Dent Res, 1989, 68(5): 773-779.
[5] Carvalho JC, Ekstrand KR, Thylstrup A. Results of 1 year of non-operative occlusal caries treatment of erupting permanent first molars. Community Dent Oral Epidemiol, 1991, 19(1): 23-28.
[6] Carvalho JC, Ekstrand KR, Thylstrup A. Results of 3 years of non-operative occlusal caries treatment of erupting permanent first molars. Community Dent Oral Epidemiol, 1992, 20(4): 187-192.
[7] Ekstrand K, Calsen O, Thylstrup A. Morphometric analysis of occlusal groove-fossa-system in mandibular third molar. Scand J Dent Res, 1991, 99(3): 196-204.
[8] Handleman S, Washburn F, Wopperer P. Two-year report of sealant effect on bacteria in dentine caries. J Am Dent Assoc, 1976, 93(5): 967-970.
[9] Handleman S. Effect of sealant placement on occlusal caries progression. Clin Prevent Dent, 1982, 4(5): 11-16.
[10] Mertz-Fairhurst E, Schuster G, Fairhurst C. Arresting caries by sealants: results of a clinical study. J Am Dent Assoc, 1986, 112(2):194-197.
[11] Braem M, Lambrechts P, Vanherle G. Stress induced cervical lesions. J Prosthet Dent, 1992, 67(5): 718-722.
[12] Lee WC, Eakle WS. Possible role of tensile stress in the etiology of cervical erosive lesions in teeth. J Prosthet Dent, 1984, 52(3): 374-380.
[13] Powell IV, Johnson GH, Gordon GE. Factors associated with clinical success of cervical abrasion/erosion restorations. Oper Dent, 1995, 20(1): 7-13.
[14] Absi EG, Addy M, Adams D. Dentin hypersensitivity. A study of the patency of dentinal tubules in sensitive and non-sensitive cervical dentin. J Clin Periodontol, 1987, 14(5): 280-284.
[15] Pashley DH. Mechanisms of dentin sensitivity. Dent Clin North Am, 1990, 34(3): 449-493.
[16] Brannstrom M. The hydrodynamics of the dentinal tubule and of pulp fluid. A discussion of its significance in relation to dentinal sensitivity. Caries Res, 1976, 1(4): 310-322.
[17] Trowbridge HO, Silver DR. A review of current approaches to in-office management of tooth hypersensivity. Dent Clin North Am, 1990, 34(3): 561-581.
[18] Tarbet WJ, Silverman G, Fratarcangelo PA, et al. Home treatment for dentinal hypersensitivity: a comparative study. J Am Dent Assoc, 1982, 105(2): 227-230.
[19] Thrash WJ, Dodds MWJ, Jones DL. The effect of stannous fluoride on dentinal hypersensitivity. Int Dent J, 1994, 44(Suppl 1): 107-118.

[20] Kim SA. Hypersensitive teeth: desensitization of pulpal sensory nerves. J Endod, 1986, 12(10): 482-485.

[21] Baume LJ, Holz J. Long term clinical assessment of direct pulp capping. Int Dent J, 1981, 31(4): 251-260.

[22] Bernick S, Nedelman C. Effect of aging on the human pulp. J Endod, 1975, 1(3): 88-94.

[23] Matsuo T, Nakanishi T, Shimizu H, et al. A clinical study of direct pulp capping applied to carious-exposed pulps. J Endod, 1996, 22(10): 551-556.

[24] Weine FS. A preview of the canal-filling materials of the 21st century. Compend Contin Educ Dent, 1992, 13(8): 688-698.

Chapter

3

Periodontal Disease

▪ Objectives

Describe the american academy of periodontology classification of periodontal disease and conditions

List clinical signs of gingival inflammation

Name and define the two major subdivisions of gingival disease

Compare and contrast dental plaque-induced gingival diseases and nonplaque-induced gingival disease

Name and define the three major categories of periodontitis

Compare and contrast chronic and aggressive periodontitis

List and describe the specific microorganisms in periodontal health, gingivitis and periodontitis

List the phases of treatment

▪ Key Concepts

Periodontal disease is a multifactorial infection elicited by a complex of bacterial species and host immune responses.

Not all gingivitis progress to periodontitis.

Additional contributing factors such as systemic conditions and local factors play a role in determining an individual's susceptibility to periodontal disease.

▪ Introduction—The Historical Background of Periodontology

Gingival and periodontal disease, in their various forms, have afflicted human since the dawn of history. Studies in paleopathology have indicated that destructive periodontal disease, as evidence by bone loss, affected early humans in such diverse cultures as ancient Egypt and early pre-Columbian America. The earliest historic records dealing with medical topics reveal an awareness of periodontal disease and the need for treatment.

Ancient Chinese also discussed periodontal disease. In the oldest book, about 2500 BC, a chapter is devoted to dental and gingival diseases. Gingival inflammations, periodontal abscess, and gingival ulceration are described. Our ancestors used the "chewstick" as a toothpick and toothbrush to clean the teeth and message the gingival tissues.

3.1   Classification of Periodontal Diseases and Conditions

3.1.1   Introduction of Disease Classification

Periodontal diseases are divided into types or classifications based on their specific bacterial etiology, development, and clinical manifestations. Gingivitis and periodontitis are two basic diagnostic categories of periodontal diseases (Figure 3-1).

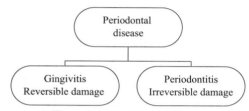

Figure 3-1   Periodontal disease
There are two major categories of periodontal diseases: gingivitis and periodontitis

Gingivitis is a bacterial infection that is confirmed to the gingiva. It results in damage to the gingival tissue that is reversible.

Periodontitis is a bacterial infection of all parts of the periodontium including the gingival, periodontal ligament, bone, and cementum. It results in irreversible destruction to the tissues of periodontium.

It is important to recognize the differences among health, gingivitis, and periodontitis (Figure 3-2).

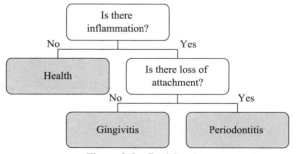

Figure 3-2   Decision tree
Is it health, gingivitis, or periodontitis

3.1.2   American Academy of Periodontology Classification System for Periodontal Diseases

Disease classification is helpful to distinguish the various conditions affecting the periodontium and to facilitate treatment planning. In periodontics, several classifications have been used, predominantly based on clinical manifestations, including location, degree of tissue change or loss, and rate of destruction. Because of a lack of understanding about specific etiology and pathogenic mechanisms, arbitrary designations have been used, such as "age" and separate "early" versus "adult" forms of disease. More recent work has suggested classification based on less subjective criteria. Additionally, despite limited microbiological and biochemical differences, the classification of the periodontal diseases has facilitated treatment alternatives and therapeutic outcomes (Table 3-1). Better understanding if the host response and the inflammation stimulated by microbial plaque should enhance the ability to distinguish periodontal diseases even more clearly.

Table 3-1   Classification of periodontal diseases and conditions

Gingival disease
    Plaque-induce gingival disease
    Non-plaque-induce gingival disease
Chronic periodontitis
    Localized
    Generalized
Aggressive periodontitis
    Localized
    Generalized
Periodontitis as a manifestation of systemic diseases

Necrotizing periodontal diseases
    Necrotizing ulcerative gingivitis (NUG)
    Necrotizing ulcerative periodontitis (NUP)
Abscesses of the periodontium
    Gingival abscess
    Periodontal abscess
    Pericoronal abscess
Periodontitis associated with endodontic lesions
    Endodontic-periodontic lesion
    Peridontic-endodontic lesion
    Combination lesion
Development or acquired deformities and conditions
    Localized tooth-related factors that predispose to plaque-induced gingival diseases or periodontics
    Mucogingival deformities and conditions around teeth
    Mucogingival deformities and conditions on edentulous ridges
    Occlusal trauma

Gingival diseases

Gingival diseases usually involve inflammation of the gingival tissues, most often in response to bacterial plaque (Table 3-2).

Table 3-2   Gingival disease

Dental Plaque-Induce Gingival Disease

These diseases may occur on a periodontium with no attachment loss or on a periodontium with attachment loss which is stable and not progressing

  I. Gingivitis associated with dental plaque only
   A. Without local contributing factors
   B. With local contributing factors
  II. Gingival diseases modified by systemic factors
   A. Associated with endocrine system
    1. Puberty-associated gingivitis
    2. Menstrual cycle-associated gingivitis
    3. Pregnancy associated
     a. Gingivitis
     b. Pyogenic granuloma
    4. Diabetes mellitus-associated gingivitis
   B. Associated with blood dyscrasias
    1. Leukemia-associated gingivitis
    2. Other
  III. Gingival diseases modified by medications
   A. Drug-influenced gingival disease
    1. Drug-influenced gingival enlargement
    2. Drug-influenced gingivitis
     a. Oral contraceptive-associated gingivitis
     b. Other
  IV. Gingival diseases modified by malnutrition
   A. Ascorbic acid deficiency gingivitis
   B. Other

Non-Plaque-Induce Gingival Lesions

  I. Gingival diseases of specific bacteria origin
   A. *Neisseria gonorrhoeae*
   B. *Treponema species*
   C. *Streptococcus species*
   D. Other

  II. Gingival diseases of viral origin
   A. Herpesvirus infections
   B. Other
  III. Gingival diseases of fungal origin
   A. Candida species infections: generalized gingival candidiasis
   B. Linear gingival erythema
   C. Histoplasmosis
  IV. Gingival lesions of genetic origin
   A. Hereditary gingival fibromatosis
   B. Other
  V. Gingival manifestations of systemic conditions
   A. Mucocutaneous lesions
    1. Lichen planus
    2. Pemphigoid
    3. Pemphigus vulgaris
    4. Erythema multiforme
    5. lupus erythematosus
    6. Drug induced
    7. Other
   B. Allergic reactions
    8. Dental restorative materials
    9. Reactions attributable to
     a. Toothpastes or dentifrices
     b. Mouth rinse or mouthwashes
     c. Chewing gum additives
     d. Foods and additives
    10. Other
  VI. Traumatic lesions (factitious, iatrogenic, or accident)
   A. Chemical injury
   B. Physical injury
   C. Thermal injury
  VII. Foreign body reaction
  VIII. Not otherwise specified

Data from Holmstrup P. Ann Periodontol, 1999 and Mariotti A. Ann Periodontol, 1999.

Periodontitis

The disease periodontitis can be subclassified into the following major three major types based on clinical, radiographic, historical, and laboratory characteristics (Table 3-3).

Table 3-3   Periodontitis

Chronic periodontitis

The following characteristics are common to patients with chronic periodontitis

- Prevalent in adults but can occur in children
- Amount of destruction consistent with local factors.
- Associated with a variable microbial pattern.
- Subgingival calculus frequently found
- Slow to moderate rate of progression with possible periods of rapid progression
- Possible modified by or associated with the following
—Systemic diseases such as diabetes mellitus and HIV infection

—Local factors predisposing to periodontitis
—Environmental factors such as cigarette smoking and emotional stress

Chronic periodontitis may be further subclassified into localized and generalized forms and characterized as slight, moderate, or severe based on the common features described above and the following specific features

- Localized form: < 30% of sites involved
- Generalized form: > 30% of sites involved
- Slight: 1 to 2 mm of clinical attachment loss
- Moderate: 3 to 4 mm of clinical attachment loss
- Severe: ≥5 mm of clinical attachment loss

Continue

Aggressive periodontitis
The following characteristics are common to patients with aggressive periodontitis
- Otherwise clinically healthy patient
- Rapid attachment loss and bone destruction
- Amount of microbial deposits inconsistent with disease severity
- Familial aggregation of diseased individuals

The following characteristic are common but not universal
- Diseased sites infected with *Aggregatibacter actinomycetemcomitans*
- Abnormalities in phagocyte function
- Hyperresponsive macrophage, producing increased prostaglandin E2 (PGE2) and interleukin-1β
- In some cases, self-arresting disease progression

Aggressive periodontitis may be further classified into localized and generalized forms based on the common features described here and following specific features
Localized form
- Circumpubertal onset of disease
- Localized first molar or incisor disease with proximal attachment loss on at least two permanent teeth, one of which is first molar
- Robust serum antibody response to infecting agents
Generalized form

- Usually affecting persons under 30 years of age (however, may be older)
- Generalized proximal attachment loss affecting at least three teeth other than fist molars and incisors
- Pronounced episodic nature of periodontal destruction
- Poor serum response to infecting agents

Periodontitis as a manifestation of systemic diseases
Periodontitis may be observed ad manifestation of the following systemic diseases
1. Hematologic disorders
   a. Acquired neutropenia
   b. Leukemia
   c. Other
2. Genetic disorders
   a. Familial and cyclic neutropenia
   b. Down syndrome
   c. Leucocyte adhesion deficiency syndromes
   d. Papillon-Lefevre syndrome
   e. Histiocytosis syndrome
   f. Glycogen storage disease
   g. Cohen syndrome
   h. hypophosphatasia
   i. Other
3. Not otherwise specified

Data from Flemming TF. Ann Periodontol, 1999 and Kinane DF. Ann Periodontol, 1999.

3. 2 Etiology and Pathogenesis of Periodontal Diseases

Gingivitis and periodontitis, as well as other less common periodontal diseases, are chronic infectious diseases. The interaction of microorganism with the host determines the course and extent of the resulting disease. Microorganisms may exert pathogenic effect directly by causing tissue destruction or indirectly by stimulating and modulating host responses. The host response is mediated by the microbial interaction and inherent characteristics of the host, including genetic factors that vary among individuals (Figure 3-3).

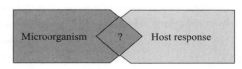

Figure 3-3   Bacteria attack vs. host response

More than 400 bacterial species are found in the human subgingival plaque samples. Of that number, possibly 10 – 20 species may play a role in the pathogenesis of destructive periodontal disease. The bacteria associated with periodontal health are primarily gram-positive facultative species and member of the genera *Streptococcus* and *Actinomyces*. Small proportion of gram-negative species are also found, most frequently *Prevotella intermedia*, *Fusobacterium nucleatum*, and *Capnocytophaga*, *Neisseria*, and *Veillonella* species. The microbiota of the dental plaque-induced gingivitis consist of approximately equal proportions of Gram-positive (56%) and Gram-negative (44%) species, as well as facultative (59%) and anaerobic (41%) microorganism. High percentages of anaerobic (90%) and gram-negative (75%) species are found from sites of chronic periodontitis. The main organisms linked with deep destructive periodontal lesions are *Porphyromonas gingivalis*, *Actinobacillus actinomycetemcomitans*, *Tannerella forsythensis*, *Treponema denticola* and *Prevotella intermedia*.

In a susceptible host, microbial virulence factors trigger the release of the host-derived enzymes and proinflammatory cytokines that can lead to periodontal tissue destruction. The implication of periodontal microbiota-associated byproducts such as endotoxin on induction of the innate immune response, toll-like receptor (TLR) signaling, generation of pathogen-associated molecular patterns (PAMPs), and their role in periodontal tissue pathogenesis are crucial to the extent of disease severity.

Elevated levels of tissue-destructive enzymes such as collagenases and other host-derived proinflammatory cytokines initiated by periodontal pathogens have been detected in inflamed gingiva and in oral fluids such as gingival crevicular fluid and saliva. In addition to antimicrobials traditionally used to manage bacterial infections in periodontitis, alternative adjunctive approaches to manage the disease target the blockade of host response modifies such as tumor necrosis factor alpha and interleukin-1 beta.

The role of host gene in the etiology and pathogenesis of periodontal diseases is critically important to the determination of patient risk for periodontal tissue breakdown. Genetic tests may prove useful for identifying patients who are most likely to develop disease, suffer from recurrent disease, it is likely that genetic test will be useful in only a subset of patients or population. Knowledge of specific genetic risk factor or inflammatory biomarkers could enable clinicians to direct environmentally based prevention and treatments to individuals who are most susceptible to disease.

3.3 Gingival Disease

The gingival tissue is constantly subjective to mechanical and bacterial aggressions. Gingival diseases are the mildest and most common form of periodontal disease.

Gingivitis is an inflammation of the gingiva causing the tissue to become red and swollen to bleed easily, and often to become slightly tender. These changes result from plaque biofilm accumulation along the gingival margins and the host's inflammatory response to the bacterial product. Gingivitis is modified by several factors such as smoking, certain drugs and hormonal changes that occur in puberty and pregnancy. Gingivitis may persist for many years without progressing to periodontitis. With good oral hygiene and effective professional removal of plaque and calculus, gingivitis is completely reversible.

3.3.1 Characteristics of Gingiva in Disease
In general, clinical features of gingivitis may be characterized by the presence of any of the following clinical signs: redness and sponginess of the gingival tissue, bleeding on provocation, changes in contour, and presence of calculus or plaque with no radiographic evidence of crestal bone loss. A systematic clinical approach requires an orderly examination of the gingival for color, contour, consistency, position, and ease and severity of bleeding and pain.

The earliest clinical symptom is gingival bleeding on probing. The absence of gingival bleeding on probing is desirable and implies a low risk of future clinical attachment loss. Interestingly, numerous studies show that current cigarette smoking suppresses the gingival inflammatory response, and smoking was found to exert a strong chronic, dose-depended suppressive effect on gingival bleeding on probing. In addition, an increase in gingival bleeding on probing in patients who quit smoking was found. Thus, people who are committed to a smoking cession program should be informed about possibility of an increase in gingival bleeding associated with smoking cession.

3.3.2 Plaque-induced Gingival Disease
Dental plaque-induced gingival are periodontal diseases involving inflammation of the gingiva in response to bacteria located at the gingival margin. There are two main subdivisions: ① plaque-induced gingivitis and ② gingival disease with modifying factors. Treatment is very effective at reversing tissue damage and returning the tissue to health.

Plaque-induced gingivitis is gingival inflammation of a periodontium resulting from dental plaque (Table 3-4).

Table 3-4 Plaque-induced gingivitis

1. Plaque present at gingival margin	6. Increased gingival exudate
2. Disease begins at the gingival margin	7. Bleeding upon provocation
3. Gingival redness, tenderness	8. Absence of attachment or bone loss
4. Swollen, rolled margins	9. Reversible with plaque removal
5. Increase in sulcular temperature	

3.3.3 Gingival Disease with Modifying Factors
There are three main subcategories of gingival disease with modifying factors: ① gingival disease modified by systemic factors (Color Figure 3-1), ② gingival disease modified by medications (Color Figure 3-2), and ③ gingival disease modified by malnutrition (see Table 3-2).

3.3.4 Nonplaque-induced Gingival Disease
A small percentage of gingival disease is not caused by bacterial plaque and does not disappear after plaque removal. It should be emphasized, however, that the presence of dental plaque could increase the

severity of the gingival inflammation in nonplaque-induced lesions. Nonplaque-induced gingivitis can result from such varied causes:

(1) Viral or fungal infections.

(2) Dermatological (skin) diseases.

(3) Allergic reactions.

(4) Mechanical trauma.

Two of these that might be seen in the dental office, primary herpetic gingivostomatitis and allergic reactions are the most common.

3. 4 Periodontitis

Periodontitis is an inflammatory disease caused by Gram negative periodontopathic bacteria, eventually leads to connective tissue destruction and alveolar bone loss. It is the result of a complex interaction between the plaque biofilm that accumulates on tooth surfaces and the body's efforts to fight this infection. Periodontitis is the number one cause of tooth loss in adults and is particularly prevalent in smoking and those who with modifying factors such as undiagnosed or poorly controlled diabetes mellitus. There are also some individuals who are genetically predisposed to developing this disease.

Periodontitis have been subdivided into three major types: ① chronic periodontitis, ② aggressive periodontitis, and ③ less common types of periodontitis.

3. 4. 1　Chronic Periodontitis—the Most Common Form

Chronic periodontitis, formally known as "adult periodontitis", is the most prevalent form of periodontitis. It is generally considered to be a slowly progressing disease. However, in the presence of systemic or environmental factors that may modify the host response to plaque accumulation, such as diabetes, smoking, or stress, disease progression may become more aggressive. Chronic periodontitis is more prevalence in adults but can also be found in children and adolescent.

Chronic periodontitis has been defined as "an infectious disease resulting in inflammation within the supporting tissues of the teeth, progressive attachment loss, and bone loss". This definition outlines the major clinical and etiologic characteristics of the disease: ① microbial plaque formation, ② periodontal inflammation, and ③ loss of attachment and alveolar bone. Periodontal pocket formation is usually a sequela of the disease process unless gingival recession accompanies attachment loss, in which case pocket depths may remain shallow, even in the presence of ongoing attachment and bone loss.

Characteristic clinical findings in patients with untreated chronic periodontitis may include supragingival and subgingival plaque accumulation (frequently associated with calculus formation), gingival inflammation, pocket formation, loss of periodontal attachment, loss of alveolar bone, and occasional suppuration (Color Figures 3-3 and 3-4).

In patients with poor oral hygiene, the gingiva typically may be slightly to moderately swollen and exhibits alternations in color ranging form pale red to magenta. Loss of gingival stippling and changes in the surface topography may include blunted or rolled gingival margins and flattened or cratered papillae.

In many patients, especially those who perform regular home care measures, the changes in color, contour, and consistency frequently associated with gingival inflammation may not be visible on inspection, and inflammation may be detected only as bleeding of the gingiva in response to examination of the periodontal pocket with a periodontal probe. The appearance of the tissue is not a reliable indicator of the presence or severity of periodontitis.

Chronic periodontitis can be clinically diagnosed by the detection of chronic inflammatory changes in the marginal gingiva, presence of periodontal pockets, and loss of attachment. It is radiographically by evidence of bone loss. These findings may be similar to those seen in aggressive periodontitis. A differential diagnosis is based on the age of the patient, rate of disease progression over time, familiar nature of aggressive disease compare with the presence of abundant plaque and calculus in chronic periodontitis.

The following characteristics are common to patients with chronic periodontitis:

Prevalent in adults but can occur in children.

Amount of destruction consistent with local factors.

Associated with a variable microbial pattern.

Subgingival calculus frequently found.

Slow to moderate rate of progression with possible periods of rapid progression.

Possible modified by or associated with the following:

Systemic diseases such as diabetes mellitus and HIV infection.

Local factors predisposing to periodontitis.

Environmental factors such as cigarette smoking and emotional stress.

Chronic periodontitis may be further subclassified into **localized** and **generalized** forms and characterized as **slight, moderate,** or **severe** based on the common features described above and the following specific features:

(1) Localized periodontitis

Periodontitis is considered localized when less than 30% of sites assessed in the mouth demonstrate attachment loss and bone loss.

(2) Generalized periodontitis

Periodontitis is considered generalized when more than 30% of sites assessed in the mouth demonstrate attachment loss and bone loss.

(3) Slight (mild) periodontitis

Periodontal destruction is generally considered slight when no more than 1 to 2 mm of clinical attachment loss has occurred.

(4) Moderate periodontitis

Periodontal destruction is generally considered moderate when 3 to 4 mm of clinical attachment loss has occurred.

(5) Severe periodontitis

Periodontal destruction is generally considered severe when 5 mm or more of clinical attachment loss has occurred.

Chronic periodontitis is generally slowly progressive, with some patients have increased susceptibility to bone loss and pocketing. Some patients who have a genetic profile that accentuates interleukin-1 production have a 2.9 times increased risk of tooth loss, and if these patients also smokers, their risk increases to 7.7 times. Diabetes is another fact that often leads to severe and extensive periodontal destruction. Also, a specific group of microorganisms is seen in the subgingival biofilm of patients ongoing bone loss associated with chronic periodontitis, including *Porphyromans gingivalis*, *Tannerella forsythensis*, and *Treponema denticola*.

3.4.2 Aggressive Periodontitis—Highly Destructive Form

Aggressive periodontitis generally affects systemically health individuals less than 30 years old, although patients may be older. Aggressive periodontitis may be universally distinguished from chronic **periodontitis** by the age of onset, the rapid rate of disease progression, the nature and composition of the associated subgingival microflora, alternations in the host's immune response, and a familiar aggregation of diseased individuals. In addition, a strong racial influence is observed in the United States; the disease is more prevalent among African Americans.

Aggressive periodontitis can be either **localized,** with first molars and incisors usually involved at or around puberty, or **generalized,** affecting at least three permanent teeth other than first molars or incisors, generally seen in patients under 30 years of age. The localized form may show decreased destructive activity when the patients are in 20s. The exact etiology for these aggressive forms of periodontitis is not known, although some patients have decreased function of polymorphonuclear leukocytes (PMNs). Several microorganisms also are suspected as playing a role, particularly *Aggregatibacter actinomycetemcomitans*, and an as-yet undetected genetic predisposition may exist as well.

Vertical loss of alveolar bone around the first molars and incisors, beginning around puberty in otherwise healthy teenagers, is a classic diagnostic sign of localized aggressive periodontitis (LAP). Radiographic findings may include and "arc-shaped" loss of alveolar bone extending from the distal surface of the second premolar to the mesial surface of the second molar. Bone defects usually wider than usually seen with chronic periodontitis (Color Figure 3-5).

A striking feature of LAP is the lack of clinical inflammation despite the presence of deep periodontal pockets and advance bone loss. Furthermore, in many cases the amount of plaque on the affected teeth is minimal, which seems inconsistent with the amount of periodontal destruction present. Evidence suggests that the rate of bone loss in LAP is three to four times faster than in chronic periodontitis. Other clinical features of LAP may include ① distolabial migration of the maxillary incisors with concomitant diastema formation, ② increasing mobility of the maxillary and mandibular incisors and first molar, ③ sensitivity of denuded root surfaces to thermal and tactile stimuli, and ④ deep, dull, radiating pain during mastication, probably caused by irritation of the supporting structures by mobile teeth and impacted food.

Clinically, generalized aggressive periodontitis (GAP) is characterized by "generalized interproximal attachment loss affecting at least three permanent teeth other than first molars or incisors". As seen in LAP, patients with GAP often have small a-mounts of bacterial plaque associated with the affected teeth. Quantitatively, the amount of plaque seems inconsistent with the amount of periodontal destruction. Qualitatively, *P. gingivalis*, *A. actinomycetemcomitans*, and *T. forsythensis* frequently are detected in the plaque that is present.

The radiographic picture in GAP can range from severe bone loss associated with the minimal number of teeth to advanced bone loss affecting the majority of teeth in the dentition. Page et al. described sites in GAP patients that demonstrated osseous destruction of 25% to 60% during a 9-week period. Despite this extreme loss, other sites in the same patient showed no bone loss.

3.5   Treatment of Periodontal Disease

Gingivitis and periodontitis are elicited primarily by bacteria. As a consequence, the treatment must have a primarily anti-infectious nature. Reduction or elimination of the infection results for the most part from mechanical treatment of affected teeth and root surfaces as well as the gingival soft tissue. In special cases, support via topical or systemic medications may be indicated. Alterable risk factors must be eliminated as much as possible.

Total treatment requires consideration of systemic aspects, including the possibility of interaction of periodontal disease with other diseases, systemic adjuncts to local treatment, and special precautions in patient management necessitated by systemic conditions. It may also entail consideration of function aspects for the establishment of optimal occlusion relationships for the entire dentition.

All these aspects are embodied in a master plan, which consists of a rational sequence of dental procedures that includes periodontal and other measures necessary to create a well-functioning dentition in a healthy periodontal environment.

The phases of treatment are summarized in Table 3-5.

Table 3-5   Phases of periodontal therapy

Preliminary phase	Rechecking
Treatment of emergency	• Pocket depth and gingival inflammation
• Dental or periapical	• Plaque and calculus, caries
• Periodontal	**Surgical phase**
• Other	Periodontal therapy, including placement of implants
Extraction of hopeless teeth and provisional replacement if needed	Endodontic therapy
Nonsurgical phase	**Restorative phase**
Plaque control and patient education	Final restorations
• Diet control (in patients with rampant caries)	Fixed and removable prosthodontic appliances
• Removal of calculus and root planning	Evaluation of response to restorative procedures
• Correction of restorative and prosthetic irritational factors	Periodontal examination
• Excavation of caries and restoration	**Maintenance phase**
• Antimicrobial therapy (local or systemic)	Periodic rechecking
• Occlusal therapy	• Plaque and calculus
• Minor orthodontic movement	• Gingival condition (pocket, inflammation)
• Provisional splinting and prosthesis	• Occlusion, tooth mobility
Evaluation of response to nonsurgical phase	• Other pathologic

In principle, the course of periodontitis therapy is similar for all forms of the disease, and is administered in stage or phase of varying duration, depending upon the extent and severity of the disease.

However, the details of individual therapy may be dramatically different. These details are dependent upon the type of disease, the patient's own desires, patient age, financial circumstances and not least, the preference of the individual clinician!

▪ Summary

Gingival diseases are the mildest form of periodontal disease. Plaque-induced gingivitis is the most common of the periodontal disease. Clinically, plaque-induced gingivitis is characterized by gingival that is red, swollen, bleeds easily, and is slightly tender. Plaque-induced gingivitis may be modified by systemic factors, medications, or malnutrition. Nonplaque-induced gingival lesions are a group of uncommon gingival lesions that are not caused by bacterial plaque. Non-plaque-induced gingivitis can result from such diverse causes as infection, skin diseases, allergic reaction, or trauma.

Periodontitis is an inflammatory disease caused by Gram negative periodontopathic bacteria, eventually leads to connective tissue destruction and alveolar bone loss. The desired outcome of periodontal therapy is to stop the progression of the disease to prevent further attachment loss. It is impossible to achieve total freedom from plaque, either supragingival or subgingivally. Therefore, the goal of periodontal therapy is to create a homeostatic balance between resident bacteria and the host response. The goal of periodontal therapy for periodontitis is firstly the complete healing of the inflammatory condition; secondly the regeneration of all lost periodontal structures.

■ Questions

1. Which of the following is a classification of periodontal disease that is described as a group of periodontal diseases that are associated with hematological disorders and genetic disorders?
   A. Chronic periodontitis
   B. Aggressive periodontitis
   C. Periodontitis as a manifestation of systemic disease
   D. Necrotizing periodontal disease

2. Which of the following is a classification of periodontal disease that is described as the most common form of periodontal disease due to inflammation of only the gingiva in response to bacteria?
   A. Gingivitis associated with dental plaque only
   B. Gingival disease modified by medication
   C. Chronic periodontitis
   D. Aggressive periodontitis

3. Over signs of inflammation include color, contour, and
   A. Purulence
   B. Alveolar bone loss
   C. Consistency

4. In gingivitis, the position of the gingival margin is
   A. Coronal to CEJ
   B. Apical to CEJ
   C. May be coronal or apical to CEJ

5. Red gingiva with multiple vesicles that easily rupture from painful ulcers is defined as:
   A. Ascorbic acid deficiency gingivitis
   B. Primary herpetic gingivostomatitis
   C. Diabetes-associated gingivitis
   D. Leukemia-associated gingivitis

6. A bacterial infection of the periodontium characterized by a rapid attachment and bone loss, high risk for tooth loss is termed:
   A. chronic periodontitis
   B. aggressive periodontitis
   C. necrotizing periodontitis

7. Tissue destruction that is characterized by probing depth of 4 to 6 mm with clinical attachment loss of up to 4 mm is termed:
   A. Advanced tissue destruction
   B. Slight to moderate tissue destruction

(**Dongqing Wang** 王冬青)

References

[1] Holmstrup P. Non-plaque-induced gingival lesions. Ann Periodontol, 1999, 4(1):20-29.
[2] Mariotti A. Dental plaque-induced gingival diseases. Ann Periodontol, 1999, 4(1): 7-17.
[3] Flemmig TF. Periodontitis. Ann Periodontol, 1999, 4(1): 32-38.
[4] Kinane DF. Periodontitis modified by systemic factors. Ann Periodontol, 1999, 4(1): 54-63.
[5] Socransky S, Haffajee A. Evidence of bacterial aetiology: a historical perspective. Periodontol, 2000, 1994, 5(1): 7-25.
[6] Zambon JJ. Periodontal diseases: microbial factors. Ann Periodontol, 1996, 1(1): 879-925.
[7] American Academy of Periodontology. Parameter on plaque induced gingivitis. J Periodontol, 2000, 71(5-s): 851-856.
[8] Dietrich T, Bernimoulin JP, Glynn RJ. The effect of cigarette smoking on gingival bleeding. J Periodontol, 2004,

75(1): 16-22.

[9] Nair P, Sutherland G, Plamer RM, et al. Gingival bleeding on probing increases after quiting smoking. J Clin Periodontol, 2003, 30(5): 435-437.

[10] Hart TC. Genetic risk factor for early-onset periodontitis. J Periodontol, 1996, 67 (4): 355-366.

[11] Loe H, Brown LJ. Early-onset periodontitis in the United State of America. J Periodontol, 1991, 62(10): 608-616.

[12] Lang N. Consensus report: aggressive periodontitis. Ann Periodontol, 1999, 4 (1): 53-53.

[13] Miller SC. Precocious advanced alveolar atrophy. J Periodontol, 1948, 19(4): 146-146.

[14] Baer JJ. The case of periodontosis as a clinical entity. J Periodontol, 1971, 42(8):516-520.

[15] Maurizio S Tonetti, Andrea Mombelli. Early-onset periodontitis. Ann Periodontol, 1999, 4 (1): 39-52.

Chapter 4

Recurrent Aphthous Stomatitis

▪ Objectives

Master recurrent aphthous stomatitis typical clinical classification, clinical features, treatment principles and commonly used drugs.

Familiar with the diagnosis and treatment.

Understanding the etiology and differential diagnosis.

▪ Key concepts

Recurrent aphthous stomatitis is the most common condition in which recurring ovoid or round ulcers affect the oral mucosa. The etiology for RAS remains unknown; but is probably multifactorial. There is no cure for RAS. Appropriate treatment depends on the degree of systemic involvement, severity of symptoms, and duration.

▪ Introduction

Recurrent aphthous stomatitis (RAS) is the most common condition in which recurring ovoid or round ulcers affect the oral mucosa. It is one of the most painful oral mucosal inflammatory ulcerative conditions and can cause pain on eating, swallowing and speaking.

4.1 Epidemiology

Epidemiological studies show an average prevalence between 15% and 50%. RAS tend to afflict women more than men and people less than 40 years. The frequency of RAS varies from less than 4 episodes per year (85% of all cases) to more than one episode per month (10% of all cases) including people suffering from continuous RAS.

4.2 Etiopathogenesis

The etiology for RAS remains unknown, but is probably multifactorial. The physical trauma, immune system reactions, genetic factors, microbiologic, nutritional have been proposed. Stress, lack of sleep, may also be a predisposing agent.

(1) Trauma to the mouth is the most common trigger. Physical trauma, such as that caused by toothbrush abrasions, laceration with sharp or abrasive foods, accidental biting, after losing teeth, or dental braces can cause aphthous ulcers by breaking the mucous membrane. Other factors, such as chemical irritants or thermal injury, may also lead to the development of ulcers.

(2) The pathogenesis of RAS involves a predominantly cell-mediated immune response in which tumor necrosis factor, or TNF, plays a major role. The immunopathogenesis probably involves cell-mediated responses, involving T cells and TNF-production by these and other leukocytes. Other cytokines such as interleukin, or IL-2, IL-10, and natural killer, or NK, cells activated by IL-2 play a role in RAS.

(3) There often is a genetic basis for RAS. More than 42% of patients with RAS have first-degree relatives with RAS. The likelihood of RAS is 90% when both parents are affected. It also is likely to be more severe and to start at an earlier age in patients with a positive family history than in those without.

(4) Hormonal imbalance. There are a few patients whose RAS remits with oral contraceptives or during pregnancy.

(5) Stress can provoke episodes of RAS, but the association is not invariable.

(6) Deficiencies in vitamin B_{12}, iron, and folic acid may contribute to RAS development. Zinc deficiency has been reported in people with RAS.

4.3 Clinical Features

There are three general forms of RAS: minor, major, and herpetiform. All are considered to be part of the same disease spectrum. Differences tend to be clinical in nature and correspond with the degree of severity. RAS are classified according to the diameter of the lesion.

4.3.1 Minor Aphthous Ulcers

Minor aphthous ulcers indicate that the lesion size is between 3 – 10 mm (Color Figure 4-1). The ulcer is covered by a yellow fibrinous membrane and surrounded by an erythematous halo. Extreme pain affecting quality of life is the obvious characteristic of the lesion. When the ulcer is white or grayish, the ulcer will be extremely painful and the affected lip may swell. They may last about 7 to 10 days without scarring. Minor RAS may present as single or multiple lesions. Minor aphthae account for 75 to 85 percent of all cases of RAS.

4.3.2 Major Aphthous Ulcers

Major aphthous ulcers have the same appearance as minor ulcerations, but are greater than 10 mm (Color Figure 4-2) in diameter and are extremely painful. They usually take more than a month to heal, and frequently leave a scar. These typically develop after puberty with frequent recurrences. They occur on movable non-keratinizing oral surfaces, but the ulcer borders may extend onto keratinized surfaces. They may last about 10 to 14 days.

4.3.3 Herpetiform Ulcers

Constituting only 5 to 10 percent of all RAS cases, herpetiform ulcers are rare. Multiple 1- to 3-mm (Color Figure 4-3). crops of small, rounded, painful ulcers resembling ulcers of herpes simplex are seen anywhere on the mucosa. They tend to fuse and produce much larger ulcers lasting 10 to 14 days. The herpetiform type of RAS presents as multiple small ulcers that tend to coalesce. Unlike herpes infections, these ulcers are not preceded by vesicles and do not demonstrate virus-infected cells.

4.4 Diagnosis

Typically, laboratory tests or biopsies are not indicated for the diagnosis of RAS. The diagnosis is often based on the clinical presentation, signs and symptoms, the recurrent nature of the problem, and the rate of healing.

4.5 Differential Diagnosis

The differential diagnosis for RAS includes traumatic ulceration, oral herpes, Behcet's syndrome, Reiter's syndrome, Crohn's disease. It is helpful to note whether the ulcers occur anywhere else in the body or if there are intestinal symptoms associated with the ulcerative condition.

(1) Traumatic ulcers are sore, painful to touch, and tend to have an irregular border erythematous margins and a yellow base. Common causes of mechanical trauma are sharp broken down teeth orthodontic and prosthetic appliances.

(2) Distinguishing RAS from recurrent oral herpes can be done based on the history of vesicles preceding ulcers, location of lesions (herpes may present both extraorally and intraorally), and laboratory studies to identify HSV.

(3) Behcet's syndrome manifests with classical RAS and a range of systemic complications, notably affecting the eyes, joints, neurological system and skin.

(4) Crohn's disease and ulcerative colitis also may occasionally be accompanied by RAS or other mouth ulcers.

4.6 Treatment

There is no conclusive evidence regarding the etiopathogenesis of recurrent aphthous stomatitis, so therapy can attempt only to suppress symptoms. Treatment aims to ease the pain when ulcers occur, and to help them to heal as quickly as possible. There is no treatment that prevents RAS from recurring. Treatment is symptomatic, the goal being to decrease symptoms; reduce ulcer number and size, and increase disease-free periods. The best treatment is that which will control ulcers for the longest period with minimal adverse side effects. The treatment approach should be determined by disease severity, the patient's medical history, the frequency of flare-ups and the patient's ability to tolerate the medication. In all patients with RAS, it is important to rule out predisposing factors and treat any such factors, where possible, before introducing more specific therapy.

4.6.1 Topical Treatment

In patients with poor oral hygiene, professional help from a dental hygienist should be considered once ulcers heal.

A number of different treatments exist for aphthous ulcers including: analgesics, anesthetics agents, antiseptics, anti-inflammatory agents, steroids.

Topical steroids, when used for a short period,

have a very safe profile and should be the first line of treatment for recurrent oral stomatitis. In addition, oral medicine specialists may administer intralesional injections of a corticosteroid such as betamethasone, dexamethasone or triamcinolone to enhance or boost the local response, thus allowing for shorter systemic treatment.

Topical application of 5% amlexanox oral paste has been shown to increase the healing rate and provide greater pain relief.

Those that exist showed that chlorhexidine gluconate mouthwashes and topical corticosteroids both can reduce the severity and duration of RAS.

4.6.2 Systemic Treatment

Patients with systemic diseases and nutritional deficiencies should be referred to appropriate health-care specialists.

In the majority of patients, symptomatic relief of RAS can be achieved with topical corticosteroids alone, with other immunomodulatory topical agents or by combination therapy. For those patients who present with major and herpetiform RAS, local and/or systemic corticosteroids, antibiotics, antiviral, and oral suspensions of tetracycline or nystatin have been recommended. In patients with recalcitrant RAS, a short course of systemic corticosteroid therapy may be required, never exceeding more than 50 mg per day (preferably in the morning) for five days. This course of treatment is best left to a physician or oral medicine specialist. If corticosteroids are used, patients should be monitored for yeast superinfection.

Its ethiopathogenesis remains unknown, and there are no diagnostic tests available. Diagnosis, therefore, is made on clinical grounds alone. Several factors—such as trauma, diet and stress—are known to trigger the disease. The most important role of the HCP is to identify underlying precipitating factors and try to eliminate them. Furthermore, it is essential to educate the patient regarding the nature of this condition, especially the fact that RAS is not a contagious condition, as often is thought, and that it is not caused by the herpes simplex virus.

Given its painful presentation and inflammatory nature, RAS responds quite well to the use of topical or systemic anti-inflammatory drugs, particularly corticosteroids. Since the advent of high-potency topical steroids, most patients with RAS can be managed this way. However, early intervention is the key.

▪ Summary

RAS is the most common condition in which recurring ovoid or round ulcers affect the oral mucosa. The lesions are painful, clearly defined, shallow, round or oval, with a shallow necrotic center covered with a yellow-grayish pseudomembrane and surrounded by raised margins and erythematous haloes. There are three general forms of RAS: minor, major, and herpetiform. All are considered to be part of the same disease spectrum. Differences tend to be clinical in nature and correspond with the degree of severity. RAS: are classified according to the diameter of the lesion. The etiology for RAS remains unknown; but are probably multifactorial. There is no conclusive evidence regarding the etiopathogenesis of recurrent aphthous stomatitis, so therapy can attempt only to suppress symptoms. Treatment aims to ease the pain when ulcers occur, and to help them to heal as quickly as possible. In the majority of patients, symptomatic relief of RAS can be achieved with topical corticosteroids alone, with other immunomodulatory topical agents or by combination therapy.

▪ Questions

1. What is recurrent aphthous stomatitis?
2. What causes recurrent aphthous stomatitis?
3. What are the treatments for recurrent aphthous stomatitis?

(**Zheng Sun**　孙正)

References

[1] Anne Field, Lesley Longman. Tyldesley's Oral Medicine. 5th ed. New York: Oxford Medical Publication, 2003:52-60.

[2] Lewkowicz N, Lewkowicz P, Banasik M, et al. Predominance of Type 1 cytokines and decreased number of CD4(+)CD25(+high) T regulatory cells in peripheral blood of patients with recurrent aphthous ulcerations. Immunol Lett, 2005: 99 (1): 57-62.

[3] Chahine L, Sempson N, Wagoner C. The effect of sodium lauryl sulfate on recurrent aphthous ulcers: a clinical study. Compend Contin Educ Dent, 1997, 18 (12): 1238-1240.

[4] McCartan BE, Sullivan A. The association of menstrual cycle, pregnancy, and menopause with recurrent oral aphthous stomatitis: a review and critique. Obstet Gynecol, 1992, 80(3 Pt 1):455-458.

[5] Scully C. Clinical practice. Aphthous ulceration. N Engl J Med, 2006, 355 (2): 165-172.

Chapter

5

Intraoral Local Anesthesia

▪ Objectives

To understand how local anesthesia works.

To know the potency, speed of onset and duration of action of common agents.

To understand nerve block anesthesia.

To be aware of anesthesia complications.

▪ Key Concepts

Infraorbital nerve block.

Posterior-superior alveolar nerve block.

Nasopalatine nerve block.

Greater palatine nerve block.

Inferior alveolar nerve block.

Complications of local anesthesia.

▪ Introduction

The use of local anesthetics to control pain during surgery in and around the mouth is a safe and well-recognized procedure. Intraoral local anesthesia procedures require the utmost care and a specific armamentarium: an anesthetic cartridge, a sterile aspirating syringe, and a sterile, disposable, stainless steel needle. When the syringe is fully assembled, the harpoon is engaged in the rubber stopper of the glass cartridge. Aspiration is achieved by pulling back on the thumb ring, and inadvertent vascular injections in the highly vascular orofacial region are avoided. Using other instruments and techniques can lead to unnecessary quantities of medication and severe adverse reactions because of inadvertent. Intravascular injection of vasoconstrictors in the local anesthetic may depress electrical activity of the cardiovascular and central nervous system or potential sympathomimetic response. Although rare, fatalities have occurred with the use of local anesthetics. Needless to say, the patient's physical status should be assessed completely before the administration of local anesthesia, because patients with certain diseases (cardiovascular, hepatic, or renal) or those treated with certain drugs (antiarrhythmics) are particularly sensitive to the pharmacologic action of these agents. Familiarity with drug interactions is imperative to anticipate alterations in the spectrum of activity of local anesthetics and individual patient response.

5.1   Types of Oral Local Anesthetics

The ideal local anesthetic is sterile, soluble in water, stable in solution, rapid in onset, completely reversible, sufficiently potent, readily metabolized, relatively nontoxic, and nonaddictive. It also has minimal adverse effects, satisfactory duration of action, and versatility. The local anesthetic agents currently available may be divided conveniently into three categories based on their relative duration of action. Procaine has a relatively short duration of action (approximately 1 hour). Mepivacaine, lidocaine, and prilocaine are of intermediate duration, and bupivacaine and etidocaine produce anesthesia of long duration. An intermediate-acting anesthetic, such as lidocaine with a vasoconstrictor, produces an average duration of soft-tissue anesthesia of approximately 2.5 hours. Long-acting local anesthetic agents with a vasoconstrictor may be most useful for the long-term relief (up to 10 hours) of acute dentoalveolar pain treated in the emergency department and for the management of postsurgical pain associated with fractures.

Procaine

Procaine hydrochloride 2-diethylaminoethyl 4-amino benzoate hydrochloride (2% solution without vasoconstrictor or with epinephrine) is an effective ester-type local anesthetic agent rapidly absorbed from injection sites. It causes local vasodilation and has a short duration of action unless it is used in conjunction with a vasoconstrictor. Procaine has limited powers of tissue penetration and is nonmyotoxic. The drug is hydrolyzed rapidly in the circulation and is excreted in the urine. It is associated with a high incidence of allergic reactions, and its use should be reserved for the patient who is truly hypersensitive to amide anesthetics. Procaine can antagonize the action of aminosalicylic acid and sulfonamides and conjugate with other drugs, prolonging their action. Death after toxic doses is usually caused by respiratory collapse. In the last 30 years, procaine has been replaced by the safer and more efficient amide local

anesthetics. It remains, however, the standard by which all new local anesthetics are evaluated and rated. In the cartridge form, it is available for use only in combination with propoxycaine.

Lidocaine

Lidocaine hydrochloride acetamide, 2-(dimethylamino)-N-(2,6-dimethylphenyl) monohydrochloride 2% solution without vasoconstrictor or with 1:100,000 epinephrine is a safe and efficacious amide derivative that has become the most widely used local anesthetic agent in the world. It provides more prompt, penetrating, intense anesthesia of longer duration of action than an equal dose of procaine hydrochloride. Lidocaine produces little or no vasodilation and may be used without a vasoconstrictor. There appears to be no evidence of cross-allergenicity between lidocaine and procaine and none between lidocaine and other amide local anesthetics. Reversible, mild, myotoxic changes have been observed after intramuscular injection. Active metabolites, such as monoethylglycinexylidide, may contribute to sedation. Death after toxic doses is usually from ventricular fibrillation.

Mepivacaine

Mepivacaine hydrochloride (1-methyl-2', 6'-pipecoloxylidide hydrochloride, 3% without, or 2% with 1:20,000 levonordefrin) is a close relative of lidocaine hydrochloride but has a more rapid onset and slightly longer duration of action. It is more myotoxic than lidocaine. Its minimal vasodilating property and low toxicity have resulted in its acceptance as a clinically safe and effective alternative to lidocaine. Because mepivacaine requires less added vasoconstrictor than all other local anesthetics, this agent is the most suitable anesthetic for the patient requiring no vasoconstrictor. Mepivacaine is metabolized less rapidly than prilocaine.

Prilocaine

Prilocaine hydrochloride (2-propylamino-o-propionotoluidide hydrochloride, 4% without vasoconstrictor and with epinephrine 1:200,000) is an amide derivative that is less potent, less toxic, and less vasodilating, and has a shorter duration of action, than lidocaine. Because it is absorbed slowly, it produces satisfactory anesthesia with or without low levels of vasoconstrictor. Metabolism occurs in both the liver and the lungs, and the drug is destroyed considerably faster than lidocaine or mepivacaine. Prilocaine has no apparent advantage in routine use over lidocaine or mepivacaine, and one of its metabolites, orthotoluidine, has been implicated in causing methemoglobinemia when doses exceed 400 mg. It is moderately myotoxic.

Bupivacaine

Bupivacaine hydrochloride (1 butyl-2', 6'-pipecoloxylidide hydrochloride, 0.5% without vasoconstrictor or with epinephrine 1:200,000) is the most potent amide-type anesthetic. This long-acting homologue of mepivacaine produces prolonged, consistent, postsurgical analgesia (approximately 7 hours) with or without a vasoconstrictor. Bupivacaine has a slower onset of action than mepivacaine, lidocaine, etidocaine and prilocaine and is metabolized at the slowest rate. Bupivacaine displays a relatively high tolerance for systemic toxicity and myotoxicity.

Articaine

Articaine hydrochloride is an amide local anesthetic. Articaine is used clinically as a 4 percent solution with epinephrine 1:100,000 or 1:200,000. The onset of anesthesia with articaine 4 percent with epinephrine 1:200,000 is 1.5 to 1.8 minutes for maxillary infiltration and 1.4 to 3.6 minutes for inferior alveolar nerve block. The duration of soft-tissue anesthesia is 2.25 hours for maxillary infiltration and approximately 4 hours for nerve block. The anesthetic activity of articaine/epinephrine combinations has been demonstrated to be comparable to that of other anesthetic combinations, including lidocaine/epinephrine, mepivacaine/levonordefrin and prilocaine/epinephrine. Articaine 4 percent with epinephrine 1:100,000 is a safe local anesthetic for use in clinical dentistry. Articaine can be used effectively in both adults and children. The use of articaine with epinephrine for local anesthesia is well-established in clinical dental practice in continental Europe and Canada, with more than 100 million cartridges having been sold. Articaine 4 percent with epinephrine 1:100,000 provides effective anesthesia with a low risk of toxicity that appears comparable to that of other local anesthetics.

5.2 Armamentarium

Local anesthetic cartridges are sealed with a paraffin-impregnated rubber plunger at one end that has been lubricated to allow greater ease of action during aspiration. The opposite end of the cartridge is the diaphragm, a rubber-filled compound sealed with an aluminum cap. There is no need to autoclave or disinfect the cartridge before use because the drug to be injected is sterile. The anesthetic solution, however, should be inspected closely. Expired, cloudy, discolored solutions or those containing particulate contamination should be discarded because their use enhances the likelihood of inadequate anesthesia. When ready for use, the cartridge is loaded into the breech of the syringe, the harpoon is engaged into the plunger, and the nonworking end of the needle is inserted into the diaphragm centrically. A few drops of anesthetic are dispensed to ensure proper function. Sterile, disposable 25- or 27-gauge needles (short needles measure 23 to 25 mm; long needles measure 36 to 40 mm) should be used for intraoral local anesthesia.

5.3 Precautions

Before administering local anesthesia, a preanesthetic evaluation of the patient should be performed. A sterile aspirating syringe should be used to minimize the risk for inadvertent intravascular injection. To prevent infection, a sterile needle should be used and latex gloves worn. The harpoon of the syringe should be engaged into the rubber plunger of the cartridge before inserting the needle to prevent bending the nonworking end of the needle.

Cognizance of the proper dosage of local anesthetics and the readiness for emergencies reduces the risk for severe adverse effects. To avoid high plasma levels of drugs and unwanted effects, several guidelines are outlined. Use the lowest drug dosage possible that gives effective anesthesia, remembering that an accumulation of the drug or of its active metabolites may occur after repeat doses of the anesthetic. Tolerance to evaluated blood levels varies with the size, weight, and medical status of the patient. The onset of local anesthetic toxicity often is preceded by the toxic effects produced by vasoconstrictors contained in local anesthetics. Local anesthetics with vasoconstrictor should be used with caution, and the dose should be restricted to a maximum of 0.04 mg (two cartridges) in patients with limited cardiovascular reserve and uncontrolled hyperthyroidism. Thyrotoxicosis is an absolute contraindication to the use of vasoconstrictors.

Local anesthetics should be used with caution in persons with known drug sensitivities to para-aminobenzoic acid and severe hepatic and renal disease. Ester-type anesthetics are contraindicated in patients with a true hypersensitivity to ester-type anesthetics; however, there is no known cross-sensitivity among the amide-type anesthetics. Prilocaine should be avoided in patients with methemoglobinemia, but patients susceptible to malignant hyperthermia are at no significant risk for adverse reactions after the administration of amide local anesthetics.

The safe use of local anesthetics in pregnant women, other than those in labor, has not been well established; however, many years of clinical use without adverse sequelae support their safety.

5.4 Injection Techniques

Proper technique is inherent to the safe and effective use of local anesthetics. To prevent vasovagal syncopal reactions, always recline the patient so that the feet are slightly higher than the head. The tissues should be pulled taut to penetrate the mucosa, and a few drops of solution should be injected as the needle is slowly advanced toward the target. To lessen the chance for breakage and deviation during insertion, a sufficiently large needle should be used. To avoid complications, do not change the direction of the needle during the injection, do not force the needle against resistance, and never insert the needle to the hub. The clinician should aspirate frequently and inject slowly to guard against intravascular injection, then slowly withdraw the needle and recap it using a sheath protector to protect against finger sticks. All needles should be disposed of in a sharps collector. The clinician should remember to communicate with the patient and to monitor his or her status before, during, and after the injection, and to have resuscitative equipment and emergency drugs immediately available whenever a local anesthetic is used.

5.5 Nerve Block Anesthesia

Nerve block anesthesia is associated with the injection of a local anesthetic agent into or near a peripheral nerve trunk or nerve plexus. This technique provides reliable, potent anesthesia to a large area with a comparatively smaller amount of drug and fewer needle punctures than other oral techniques. Nerve block is particularly useful for mandibular anesthesia and for anesthesia of inflamed or infected tissue when needle penetration of the infection site could result in dissemination. Nerve block anesthesia can be performed on these orofacial nerves: infraorbital, posterior superior alveolar, middle supe-

rior alveolar, anterior superior alveolar, nasopalatine, greater palatine, inferior alveolar, lingual, buccal, mental, and incisive.

5.5.1 *Infraorbital Nerve Block*

The infraorbital nerve is the terminal branch of the maxillary nerve exiting from the infraorbital foramen at the midface. It branches into the anterior superior alveolar nerve, middle superior alveolar nerve, inferior palpebral nerve, lateral nasal nerve, and superior labial nerve and supplies sensory innervation to the skin of the inferior eyelid, lateral nose, and upper lip and the mucous membrane lining the nasal vestibule. The infraorbital nerve block provides profound pulpal and labial mucosa anesthesia from the maxillary central incisor through the second premolar and is more reliable and efficient than the anterior superior alveolar and the middle superior alveolar nerve blocks. The nerve may be anesthetized from an intraoral or extraoral approach (Color Figure 5-1).

The intraoral approach uses a 36-mm, 25- or 27-gauge needle. First, locate the infraorbital notch and foramen by extraoral palpation at the mid-infraorbital ridge along a vertical line with the pupil of the eye and the first premolar. Maintain light finger pressure on the foramen, lift the upper lip, and retract the cheek laterally. Insert the needle at the crest of the mucobuccal fold directly over the first bicuspid. Advance the needle slowly, keeping it parallel with the long axis of the maxillary bicuspid. The needle should penetrate approximately 15 mm at the point of contact with the upper rim of the infraorbital foramen. Aspirate, then deposit 1. 2 to 1. 5 mL of local anesthetic solution to the foramen.

For the extraoral approach, wash and disinfect the skin covering the infraorbital foramen. Locate the infraorbital foramen as before and grasp 2 cm of soft tissue overlying the foramen between the thumb and the index finger. Direct a 23-mm, 25-gauge needle into the fold of tissue approximately 6 mm below the foramen. The approach should be from the medial, just adjacent to the thumb, and lateral to the ala of the nose. Advance the needle slowly upward, and posterior with the barrel of the syringe in proximity to the upper lip. Make gentle contact with the rim of the infraorbital foramen, then aspirate, and deposit 1. 2 to 1. 5 mL of anesthetic solution.

5.5.2 *Posterior-superior Alveolar Nerve Block*

The posterior-superior alveolar nerve is blocked by

injecting local anesthetic behind the infrazygomatic crest and immediately distal to the second molar tooth. Anesthesia of the facial mucoperiosteum and the pulp of the maxillary molar teeth, excluding the mesiobuccal root of the first molar, is obtained. A 25-mm, 25- or 27-gauge needle is inserted at the depth of the second and third molar mucobuccal fold. The needle is advanced upward, inward, and posteriorly along the distal surface of the maxillary tuberosity where the posterior-superior alveolar nerve enters the maxilla. To ensure success, the needle should remain in close contact with the tuberosity. The final depth of penetration is approximately 1.5 cm (Color Figure 5-2). The need for aspiration is great because this is a significant location for hematoma.

5.5.3   Nasopalatine Nerve Block

The nasopalatine nerve supplies sensory innervation to the soft tissues of the anterior third of the palate. To anesthetize this nerve, a 27-gauge needle is inserted through the lateral aspect of the incisive papillae located along the mid-palatal raphe, 2 mm posterior to the maxillary central incisors. With the mouth open fully, the barrel of the syringe parallels the long axis of the maxillary incisors and is in close contact with the mandibular incisors. As the needle is slowly advanced toward the incisive canal, a few tenths of a milliliter is deposited. The needle need not be inserted beyond a penetration depth of 3 mm to achieve adequate anesthesia. In addition, because the mucoperiosteum of the palate in this location is taut, less than 0.3 mL should be delivered. Topical anesthetic is particularly useful for this injection. Overlapping innervation from the greater palatine nerve in the cuspid region may require additional anesthesia if profound anesthesia of the cuspid area is required (Color Figure 5-3).

5.5.4   Greater Palatine Nerve Block

The greater palatine nerve innervates the posterior two thirds of the hard palate and part of the soft palate. A 27-gauge short needle is used to anesthetize this nerve. The needle is directed from the anterior oral cavity toward the third molar region along the palatal vault.

With the bevel toward bone, the penetration site of the needle is 0.7 to 1 cm medial and superior to the maxillary second molar. A few drops of anesthetic solution are deposited as the needle is ad-

vanced slowly toward the greater palatine foramen. At a depth of approximately 4 mm, the palatine bone is contacted gently, the needle is withdrawn slightly, and aspiration performed. Blanching of the soft tissue occurs as 0.3 to 0.5 mL of local anesthetic solution is deposited under the palatal mucosa. Soft-tissue anesthesia anteriorly to the first bicuspid and medially to the midline is achieved within several minutes (Color Figure 5-4).

5.5.5   Inferior Alveolar Nerve Block

Successful anesthesia of the mandibular arch requires precise nerve block anesthesia because diffusion of solution during infiltration is thwarted by the thickness and density of the mandibular cortical plate. Mastery of this nerve block is challenged by the small target area, large distance over which the needle must travel, and limited diffusion of agent that occurs when the solution is deposited erroneously. The inferior alveolar nerve block, when properly performed, provides unilateral anesthesia to the inferior alveolar nerve, mental nerve, and incisive nerve, which innervate the ipsilateral mandibular teeth, mucous membranes, periodontal structures, and the body of the mandible anterior to the mandibular foramen. Frequently, the lingual nerve is anesthetized by this nerve block during withdrawal of the needle after the inferior alveolar nerve block has been performed (Color Figure 5-5). The intraoral method for the right inferior alveolar nerve block is described below.

The inferior alveolar nerve is approached from the anterior aspect, and the solution is ultimately deposited in the pterygomandibular space near the medial surface of the ramus, just before the nerve enters the mandibular foramen. Mental visualization of the nerve's location is the first step in the procedure. The patient's mouth should be opened fully, and the patient should be advised to maintain this position until the injection is complete. The mucobuccal fold is retracted with the thumb of the noninjecting hand, and the greatest curvature of the ascending ramus (coronoid notch) and the internal oblique ridge is palpated. While maintaining the thumb's intraoral position, determine the width of the mandible by grasping the posterior border of the mandibular ramus with the first phalanx. The mandibular foramen is visualized mentally as the midpoint along an imaginary line between the thumb and the first digit. The anteroposterior and inferosuperi-

or position of the mandibular foramen also can be judged from a panoramic radiograph.

The buccal tissues are retracted laterally, and the V-shaped pterygotemporal depression is exposed between the pterygomandibular raphe and the internal oblique ridge. A 36-mm, 25-gauge needle is inserted lateral to the pterygomandibular raphe through the mucosa of the pterygotemporal depression along a line that parallels the occlusal plane approximately 1 cm above the occlusal surface of the third molar. As the needle is advanced toward the mandibular sulcus, the barrel of the syringe should be located over the contralateral bicuspids to ensure that the needle parallels the flared inner aspect of the ramus. A few drops of anesthetic solution are deposited during passage of the needle through the buccopharyngeal fascia and the buccinator muscle to minimize discomfort. The needle is advanced in a straight path for 1. 5 to 2 cm (two thirds the length of a long needle), where gentle contact with the periosteum occurs. The depth of needle insertion may vary according to the size of the patient; however, depths less than 1 cm or greater than 2. 5 cm often indicate incorrect needle location. The needle is withdrawn slightly to avoid subperiosteal injection. The clinician then aspirates and slowly deposits 1. 2 to 1. 8 mL of solution at, or near, the mandibular foramen over a 1-minute period. No greater solution is needed for intraoral anesthesia because the maximum volume of the pterygomandibular space is approximately 2 mL. The proximity of the lingual nerve to the inferior alveolar nerve in this region often results in complementary lingual anesthesia. Anesthesia may be incomplete on the buccal aspect of the molar region because of innervation by the long buccal nerve.

5. 6   Adverse Effects

Local anesthetics are safe drugs with a wide therapeutic index, yet complications may arise despite careful attention to proper technique. For the most part, untoward reactions are the direct consequence of the pharmacologic properties of the agent, the presence of a vasoconstrictor or other additive, rapid systemic absorption, concomitant drug therapy, and vasovagal response, with psychogenic reactions the most common. Other adverse experiences include idiosyncratic reactions, diminished patient tolerance, immediate blanching of the facial skin, deviation of the eye and transient blurring or loss of vision, facial

nerve palsy, hematoma formation, and hypersensitivity reactions such as angioedema, urticaria, dermatitis, or anaphylaxis. Usually hypersensitivity is attributed to methylparaben, a bacteriostatic and fungistatic preservative included in multiple-dose vials. Tissue sloughing, myositis, parasthesia, and postinjection pain may occur if excessive amounts of local anesthetic solution are deposited or if the needle damages a nerve during the injection. Recurrent herpes simplex is a common postanesthetic lesion.

Serious adverse reactions, generally systemic in nature, result directly from the amount and rate of drug dose and drug absorption relative to drug elimination. Rapid absorption caused by a too-rapid injection, inadvertent intravascular injection, or injection into a highly vascular area are common causes. Other causes include altered detoxification, administration of too large an amount of local anesthetic, injection of the wrong concentration, injection without a vasoconstrictor, and failure to correct for the patient's physical status. Different local anesthetics that are equally potent may differ markedly in their toxicity. The signs and symptoms of toxicity predominate in the central nervous and cardiovascular systems.

Sympathomimetic vasoconstrictors, along with the release of endogenous catecholamines, may elicit adverse effects in some patients. In healthy persons, the effect is usually transitory because the total dose of epinephrine is small. Mild side effects include heart palpitations, throbbing headache, tenseness, and tremor. In patients with chronic cardiovascular disease, severe reactions may cause cardiac arrhythmias, chest pain, or cardiac arrest. Because of these effects, vasoconstrictors should be used with caution in patients with hyperthyroidism, pheochromocytoma, cardiovascular disease, and recent myocardial infarction. In addition, long-acting anesthetics, such as etidocaine and bupivacaine, have more cardiac depressant properties than lidocaine. Deaths have been documented after caudal anesthesia using long-acting anesthetics.

Hypersensitivity reactions to local intraoral anesthesia are rare. When they occur, urticaria and difficulty in breathing are the first clinical manifestations. If the symptoms progress to anaphylaxis, immediate action is required. Epinephrine (0. 5 mL of a 1 : 1000 solution) delivered into the floor of the mouth or subcutaneously, followed by oxygen, Benadryl, intravenous access, and hydrocortisone, is indicated.

▪ Summary

1. Common local anaesthetic drugs include mepivacaine, lidocaine, prilocaine, bupivacaine and etidocaine.

2. General complications of local anaesthesia are psychogenic, toxic and allergy.

3. Local complications of local anaesthesia are soft-tissue trauma, nerve, trauma and intravacular injection.

▪ Questions

1. Which anesthetic methods should be used in extraction of maxillary premolars?

2. Which anesthetic methods should be applied in extraction of mandibular molars?

3. What complications can occur after local anaesthesia?

(Jingming Liu   刘静明)

References

[1] Stanley F malamed. Handbook of local anesthesia. 5th ed. Singapore: Elsevier, 2006: 66-99, 225-313.

[2] Stanley F malamed, Suzanne Gagnon, Dominique leblanc. Articaine hydrochloride: a study of the safety of a new amide local anesthetic. J Am Dent Assoc, 2001, 132(2):177-185.

Chapter 6

Dental Extractions

▪ Objectives

To understand the indication and contraindications for removal of a tooth.

To know the techniques available for extraction.

To be aware of the potential complications following extraction and their treatment.

▪ Key Concepts

Indication, contraindications and complications of dental extraction

▪ Introduction

In this chapter, the surgical treatment of teeth is described. The indications and contraindications for dental extraction are listed together with the information that must be elicited before a tooth is extracted. Forceps and surgical techniques of extraction are outlined and the complications that can follow extraction are outlined with the treatment response.

6.1 Indications for the Extraction of Teeth

(1) Teeth that are hopelessly carious.

(2) Teeth with nonvital pulps, or acute or chronic pulpitis when root canal surgery is not indicated.

(3) In cases of severe periodontoclasia in which excessive bony support of the teeth is destroyed.

(4) Teeth not treatable by apicoectomy.

(5) Teeth mechanically interfering with the placement of restorative appliances.

(6) Teeth not restorable by operative dentistry.

(7) Impacted teeth and unerupted teeth.

(8) Supernumerary teeth.

(9) Retained primary teeth when a permanent tooth is present,

and in normal position to erupt.

(10) Teeth with fractured roots.

(11) Malposed teeth not amenable to orthodontic treatment.

(12) Roots and fragments.

(13) Teeth that are traumatizing soft tissues, if other treatment will not prevent this trauma.

6.2 Contraindications for the Extraction of Teeth

Contraindications to the extraction of teeth before any oral surgical procedure, including the removal of teeth, is undertaken, a thorough oral examination and physical survey of the patient is mandatory.

6.2.1 Systemic Contraindications

6.2.1.1 Cardiac disease

(1) Breathlessness is one of the first and most reliable signs of cardiac disease.

(2) Chronic fatigue is a frequent indication of heart failure.

(3) Palpitation of recent origin, induced now by activities which heretofore were tolerated without fatigue.

(4) Sleep which is disturbed unless the head is elevated.

(5) Headache from cerebral congestion.

(6) Vertigo from relative cerebral anemia.

(7) Cyanosis of the lips, tongue or fingernails.

(8) Dyspnea on exertion.

(9) Engorged cervical veins.

(10) Edema of the ankles.

(11) Exophthalmos, with goiter, nervousness or sweating.

(12) Tachycardia, pulse markedly accelerated.

(13) Petechiae in the mouth or elsewhere.

(14) Blood pressure within normal limits.

6.2.1.2 Blood dyscrasias

(1) Anemia.

(2) Leukemia.

(3) Hemorrhagic purpura.

(4) Hemophilia.

6.2.1.3 Diabetes

Uncontrolled diabetes is a contraindication to oral surgery, because this disease predisposes to the development of infection in the wound with extension into the surrounding tissues.

6.2.1.4 Nephritis

If there is any indication of nephritis in a patient requiring extraction of teeth, refer the patient to his physician for diagnosis and treatment before instituting oral surgery.

6.2.1.5 Toxic goiter

A thyroid crisis may be precipitated by oral surgery. The patient with a thyroid crisis is semiconscious, very restless, uncontrollable even with heavy sedation cyanotic, and at times delirious, with an extremely rapid, thready pulse and a high temperature. No oral surgery procedure, including the extraction of teeth, should be performed on a patient with a toxic goiter, since such trauma may precipitate a crisis of thyroid activity with cardiac embarrassment and heart failure.

6.2.1.6 Syphilis

The syphilitic patient's resistance is lowered, so that he is more liable to the development of postoperative infection because of delayed healing. These patients should be on antisyphilitic treatment before oral surgery is performed.

6.2.1.7 Jaundice

The symptoms include yellowish or bronzed skin and conjunctiva, yellow mucous membranes, and yellowish body fluids. Patients with jaundice should be referred to their physicians for treatment before undergoing oral surgery.

6.2.2 Local Contraindications to the Extraction Teeth

(1) Acute gingival infection.

(2) Acute pericoronal infection.

(3) Extraction of maxillary bicuspids and molars is contraindicated during acute maxillary sinusitis.

6.3 Complications of Dental Extractions

6.3.1 Postoperative Pain

Discomfort after surgical trauma of dental extractions is to be expected and may be alleviated with an analgesic such as paracetamol or a non-steroidal anti-inflammatory drug(NSAID) such as ibuprofen. Severe pain after dental extraction is unusual and may indicate that another complication has occurred.

6.3.2 Postoperative Swelling

Mild inflammatory swelling may follow dental extractions but is unusual unless the procedure was difficult and significant surgical trauma occurred.

More significant swelling usually indicates postoperative infection or presence of a hematoma. Management of infection may require systemic antibiotics or drainage. A large hematoma may need to be drained. Less likely is surgical emphysema.

6.3.3 Trismus
Trismus or limited mouth opening after a dental extraction is unusual and is likely to be infective in origin.

6.3.4 Fracture of Teeth
Teeth may fracture during forceps extraction for a variety of reasons and this is not an unusual event. The crown may fracture because of the presence of a large restoration, but this may not prevent the extraction from continuing as the forceps are applied to the root. However, If the fracture occurs subgingivally, then a transalveolar will be necessary to visualize the root.

If a small root apex is retained after extraction, this may be left in situ, providing it is not associated with apical infection. The patient must be informed of the decision to leave the apex to avoid the morbidity associated with its surgical retrieval and the decision recorded. Antibiotics should be prescribed.

6.3.5 Excessive Bleeding
It may be difficult to gauge the seriousness of the blood loss from the patient's history, because they are usually anxious. However, it is important to establish whether or not the patient is shocked by measuring the blood pressure and pulse. This can be done while the patient bites firmly on a gauze swab to encourage haemostasis. Typically if the systolic pressure is below 100 mmHg and the heart rate in excess of 100 beats/min, then the patient is shocked and there is an urgent need to replace lost volume. This may be done by infusion of a plasma expander such as gelofusine or haemaccel or a crystalloid such as sodium chloride via a large peripheral vein. For this purpose, the patient should be transferred to hospital. More commonly, the patient is not shocked and can be managed in the primary care setting.

The next step in management is to investigate the cause of the hemorrhage by taking a history and carrying out an examination.

Determine the source of the hemorrhage by sitting the patient upright and using suction and a good light. This is commonly from capillaries of the bony socket or the gingival margin of the socket, or more unusually from a large blood vessel or soft-tissue tear.

The following technique could be used:

Socket capillaries: pack the socket with resorbable cellulose, such as sugicell.

Gingival capillaries: suture the socket with a material that will permit adequate tension, such as vicryl or black silk.

Large blood vessel: ligate vessel, usually by passing a suture about the vessel and soft tissues.

6.3.6 Dry Socket (Alveolar Osteitis)
In some cases, a blood clot may inadequately form or be broken down. Predisposing factors of osteitis include smoking. Surgical trauma, the vasoconstrictor added to a local anesthetic solution, oral contraceptives and a history of radiotherapy. The exposed bone is extremely painful and sensitive to touch.

Dry socket is managed by: ① Reassuring the patient that the correct tooth has been extraction; ② Irrigation of socket with warn saline or chlorhexidine mouthrinse to remove any debris; ③ Dressing the socket to protect it from painful stimuli: bismuth-iodoform-paraffin paste (BIPP) and lidocaine gel on ribbon gauze are useful.

6.3.7 Postoperative Infection
In some cases, sockets may become truly infected, with pus, local swelling and perhaps lymphadenopathy. This is usually localized to the socket and can be managed in the same way as a dry socket, although antibiotics may be taken to exclude the presence of a retained root or sequestered bone. Positive evidence of such material in the socket indicates a need for curettage of the socket.

6.3.8 Osteomyelitis
Osteomyelitis is rare but may be identified by radiological evidence of loss of the socket lamina dura and a rarefying osteitis in the surrounding bone, often with scattered radio-opacities representing sequestra.

6.3.9 Damage to Soft Tissues
Crush injured can occur to soft tissues when a local or general anesthetic has been used and the patient dose not respond to the stimulus and, therefore, inform the operator. This may happen to a lower anesthetized lip when extracting an upper tooth; the lip can be crushed between forceps and teeth if it is not rotated out of the way.

6.3.10   Damage to Nerves

Paraesthesia or anaesthesia can result from damage to the nerves in the intradermal canal during extraction of lower third molars.

6.3.11   Opening of the Maxillary Sinus

Creation of a communication between the oral cavity and maxillary sinus, an oroantral fistula, may result during extraction of upper molar teeth.

6.3.12   Loss of Tooth

A whole tooth may occasionally be displaced into the maxillary sinus, when it is managed as for displacement of a root fragment. A tooth may also be lost into the infratemporal fossa or the tissue spaces about the jaws, but this usually only occurs when mucoperiosteal flap raised.

6.3.13   Loss of Tooth Fragment

Typically, a fractured palatal root of an upper molar tooth is inadvertently pushed into the maxillary sinus by the misuse of elevators. Rarely, a fragment may be lost elsewhere, such as into the inferior alveolar canal.

6.3.14   Fracture of Jaw

A fracture of the jaw is a rare event and is most likely to be the result of application of excessive force in an uncontrolled way. More commonly, small fragments of alveolar bone are fractured, which may be attached to the tooth root. Any loose fragments should also be removed.

6.3.15   Dislocation of the Mandible

Dislocation may occur when extracting lower teeth if the mandible is not adequately supported. It is more likely to occur under general anaesthesia and should be reduced immediately.

6.3.16   Displacement of Tooth into the Airway

The air way is at risk when extracting teeth on a patient in the supine position. It can be protected when the patient is being treated under general anaesthesia but not when the patient is conscious or being treated under conscious sedation. It is, therefore, essential that an assistant is present and high-velocity suction and an appropriate instrument for retrieval of any foreign body are immediately available. A chest radiograph is essential if a lost tooth cannot be found, to exclude inhalation.

6.3.17   Surgical Emphysema

Air may enter soft tissues, producing a characteristic crackling sensation on palpation. However, this is unlikely if a mucoperiosteal flap has not been raised. Air-rotor dental drills should not be used during surgery because they may force air under soft-tissue flaps. The patient should be reassured and antibiotics prescribed.

6.4   Dental Extractions

Exodontia is the clinical practice of extracting teeth and tooth fragments. The ideal aim of exodontia is to remove the entire tooth with minimal trauma to surrounding tissues. In clinical practice, dental extractions can be simple intra-alveolar forceps extractions or difficult transalveolar surgical extraction.

Simple exodontia, otherwise referred to as intra-alveolar extraction, pertains to the removal of teeth from their bony alveolar sockets without the need to create a surgical pathway for the delivery of the tooth.

Surgical exodontia is the removal of teeth or tooth fragments via the transalveolar approach, whereby access to and delivery of the tooth or its fragments is achieved via a surgically created pathway. In the transalveolar approach, the alveolar bone and soft tissues surrounding the tooth or its fragments are surgically breached to create a pathway required for surgical exodontia.

6.4.1   Armamentarium for Dental Extractions

The practice of exodontia requires a variety of instruments, which may be divided into the following broad categories:

Extractors are the main instruments used to physically remove teeth and tooth fragments from their bony alveolar sockets. There are two types of extractor:

(1) Dental forceps.

(2) Dental elevators.

Nonextractors are accessory instruments used to facilitate the exodontia procedure in three ways:

(1) Access to the tooth and maintenance of a surgical field clear of blood and debris that may interfere with the direct field of vision of the operator.

(2) Removal of surrounding tissues to allow proper placement or positioning of the extraction in-

struments.

（3）Repair of the surgical wound following thorough irrigation and debridement of the remaining tooth socket.

Dental forceps

Dental forceps are the oldest and most frequently used of all surgical instruments in the practice of exodontia. There are numerous dental forceps designs and configurations, depending on the tooth to be extracted. Generally speaking, all forceps used to extract mandibular teeth have a right-angle bend between the handles and the beaks. Forceps used to extract maxillary teeth range from straight to curved to anatomical left- and right-type beak configurations. The further posterior the teeth are, the greater the curvature of the beaks required to extract the teeth.

Dental elevators

Dental elevators are the other most commonly used surgical instruments in exodontia. These instrument are particularly useful in surgical extraction. The greatest variations in the type and design of an elevator are found in the shape and size of the blade. The two basic elevators patterns are straight or curved, depending on the direction of the blade tip relative to the shank.

6. 4. 2 Simple Exodontia

The bare essentials required for simple exodontia are as follows:

（1）An informed patient.

（2）A basic examination set, including dental mirror, dental probe, tweezers, and gauze.

（3）Strong light and adequate suction.

（4）Local anesthetic, including a needle, dental syringe, and local anesthetic carpule.

（5）Dental extraction instruments: dental forceps and dental elevators.

6. 4. 3 Extraction Technique

The most effective way to extract teeth is to cultivate a technique of removing the whole tooth with minimal trauma to surrounding tissues. A good extraction technique entails two fundamental requirements:

（1）adequate access to the tooth.

（2）Use of controlled force to luxate and deliver the tooth.

Adequate access

Adequate access to the tooth is facilitated by the proper positioning of the clinician and the patient. For the greatest mechanical advantage, it is best if the clinician is standing for all extractions. Furthermore, the nondominant hand should be used to retract the lips and tongue, with fingers on either side of the alveolus, and to support the jaw.

Use of controlled force

The successful removal of teeth with forceps relies largely on the proper use of controlled force. Excessive force, particularly in awkward directions, can lead to fractures of the crown and hence increase the operating time and surgical morbidity for the patient.

Basic steps of forceps extractions

The dental forceps are the most commonly used and often the only instruments required for the simple intra-alveolar extraction of teeth. Simple forceps extractions involve the following four basic steps:

（1）Grasping of the tooth: use the beaks of the forceps to grasp the whole crown of the tooth and part of the root 1 to 2 mm beyond the cementoenamel junction.

（2）Expansion of the bony socket.

（3）Mobilization of the tooth.

（4）Delivery of the complete and intact tooth.

The following basic forces are used to expand the socket and mobilize the tooth:

（1）Apical pressure to break the periodontal seal.

（2）Buccal force to expand the buccal plate of bone.

（3）Lingual force to expand the lingual crest of bone.

（4）Rotational force, resulting in overall expansion of the tooth socket.

（5）Traction force: to deliver the tooth.

Always commence with apical pressure and end with traction force to deliver the tooth.

Forceps removal of individual teeth

The extraction technique depends on the tooth being extracted, which is in turn dictated by the morphology of the tooth and, in particular, its root anatomy. Different teeth not only require different forceps patterns but also particular extraction forces.

（1）Maxillary teeth

1）Incisors —maxillary straight forceps
—single conical root
—mainly rotational force required

2）Canines —stubby forceps

—single long root

—buccal-palatal rocking and rotational forces required

3) Premolars—maxillary universal forceps

—single or double roots that are flattened mesiodistally

—mainly buccolingual movement required

4) Molars —maxillary left and right hawk's bills(anatomic)forceps

—three conical roots splayed in a triangular configuration

—mainly buccal force required

(2) Mandibular teeth

1) Incisors —mandibular universal forceps

—single root, flattened mesiodistally

—mainly buccolingual movement required

2) Canines and premolars

—mandibular universal forceps

—single conical root

—mainly rotational force required

3) Molars —mandibular hawk's bills(anatomic) forceps

—two roots, flattened mesiodistally

—figure-eight movement with buccolingual forces required

Surgical exodontia

All dental practitioners should be conversant with the principles of surgical exodontia, which is employed for the removal of difficult erupted teeth, retained roots, and impacted teeth.

Basic steps of surgical exodontia:

(1) Flap design.

(2) Bone removal.

(3) Tooth division.

(4) Tooth or fragment removal.

(5) Wound cleaning.

(6) Primary closure.

Not all surgical extractions require each of six steps. In many cases, a tooth may be surgically extracted simply by raising a flap without having to remove bone or divide the tooth. Each of the steps will be discussed in more detail.

Flap design

A flap is a mass of tissue comprising a base and a distal segment, which is raised from its surrounding tissue bed. A flap serves two fundamental purposes.

(1) To gain access to the surgical site.

(2) To serve as the primary dressing to cover the surgical defect that is created.

Many types of flap are used in surgery, but in surgical exodontia a mucoperiosteal flap, consisting of the oral mucosa and periosteum that covers the alveolar process, is used.

Flaps may also be described in terms of their physical shape or outline or, more often, according to the site from which the flap is procured, such as buccal flap, palatal flap, lingual flap, and so on.

Technical notes:

(1) Make the incision in one continuous stroke through to bone at right angles to the surface of the mucosa.

(2) Always make the base of the flap, where the blood supply is derived, wider than its distal segment to maintain the viability of the flap when it is raised from its tissue bed.

(3) Always include the entire dental papilla on the distal margin of the flap to avoid poor gingival contours after healing.

(4) Once you raise the flap with the aid of a periosteal elevator, handle the flap gently to avoid stretching and tearing of its margins, which will compromise its healing potential.

(5) Ideally, ensure that the edges of the flap lie on sound bone at the end of the operative procedure to prevent wound dehiscence and breakdown.

Bone removal

Bone is removed to expose enough teeth to:

(1) Permit the application of dental elevators.

(2) Allow adequate exposure for sectioning of the tooth.

(3) Provide an adequate pathway for delivery of the tooth or tooth fragments.

Bone may be removed by the use of:

(1) Sharp chisels.

(2) Powered handpieces with round or fissured surgical burs that are water cooled with the exhaust facing away from the surgical site. High-speed air turbines may create a surgical wound emphysema and do not allow enough tactile discrimination between bone and tooth substance.

Tooth division

It is particularly useful to section teeth in the following cases:

(1) Where the awkward angulation and curvature of the roots of a multirooted tooth does not permit its delivery in one piece.

(2) Where smaller fragments can be easily lifted out of the bony socket, thereby minimizing the need to remove further bone.

Teeth can be sectioned in the following ways:

(1) Osteotome: this method is quick but the split is often unpredictable.

(2) Powered handpiece: this technique is slow but more predictable. The split may be completed with a straight elevator after the bur has penetrated the pulp chamber of the tooth.

Technical notes:

The direction in which teeth are divided (axial, coronal, vertical, or horizontal) depends on:

(1) the angulation of the tooth.

(2) the number and pattern of the roots.

(3) the path of delivery of the tooth or its individual fragments.

Tooth or fragment removal

This step constitutes the most important part of the whole surgical exercise. The successful removal of the tooth or tooth fragments is largely dependent on:

(1) The quality of the surgical access created, that is, whether enough bone has been removed to adequately expose the site for the application of a dental elevator.

(2) The correct use of the dental elevators, basically requiring a suitable point of purchase or fulcrum for the instrument to be used in a rotating motion to luxate the tooth or tooth roots.

Wound cleaning

After the whole tooth or all of the tooth fragments have been completely removed, the remaining surgical defect must be thoroughly debrided and irrigated to remove all loose debris that may cause infections and delay wound healing. Wound cleaning may involve:

(1) Excision of redundant soft tissue.

(2) Curettage of the base of the socket, especially following the extraction of nonvital teeth, to clear out any periapical pathosis such as a periapical granuloma or dental cyst.

(3) Removal of any loose fragments of bone or tooth in and around the surgical defect, including under the flap.

(4) Smoothing of rough bony edges with burs or bone files.

(5) Irrigation of the wound with sterile isotonic sodium chloride solution (saline) and suctioning of the area to remove microscopic debris.

(6) Occasionally, application of antibiotic pow-der or dressing with antiseptic-soaked ribbon gauze; this is a rare occurrence.

Primary closure

The surgical defect must be sealed from the oral environment by replacement of the flap and careful suturing to permit well-approximated wound margins without tension. The flap acts as the primary dressing and contains the osteogenic layer of periosteum, which will help promote bone regeneration within the surgical defect.

It is best if the tying of sutures is first demonstrated by an experienced clinician and then practiced on a rubber dam before beginning on patients. There are two methods of tying suturing:

(1) Instrument tying: the knot is established by passing the suture once (square knot) or twice (surgeon's knot) around the tip of the needle holders. The knot is tightened and then locked by passing the suture around the needle holder in the opposite direction.

(2) Hand tying: this is rarely used in exodontia.

In surgical exodontia the most common suturing pattern is the simple interrupted suture. The second most common is the horizontal mattress suture, which is used to hold together soft tissues over a tooth extraction socket.

■ Summary

Teeth may need removal for many reasons including the following: caries, pulpitis, periapical periodontitis and pericoronitis when associated with other pathology such as a cyst, fracture of jaw or tumour, misplaced, impacted or supernumerary, as part of orthodontic treatment, retained primary teeth.

Contraindications for the extraction of teeth include cardiac disease, blood dyscrasias, diabetes, nephritis, toxic goiter, syphilis, jaundice, acute gingival infection, acute pericoronal infection.

■ Questions

1. What are the complications of dental extractions and how to avoid?

2. What are the principles of surgical removal of teeth?

(**Jingming Liu**　刘静明)

References

[1] Paul Coulthard, Philip Sloan, Keith Horner, et al. Oral and maxillofacial surgery, radiology, pathology and oral medicine. 2nd ed. Beijing: Peking University Medical Press, 2009: 87-91.

[2] Dimitroulis George. Illustrated lecture notes in oral and maxillofacial surgery. China: Quintessence Publications Co. , 2008: 35-49.

[3] Archer William Harry. Oral and maxillofacial surgery. 5th ed. Philadelphia: W. B. Saunders company, 1975: 15-22.

Chapter 7

Infection and Inflammation of the Tooth and Jaws

▪ Objectives

Recognize the symptoms and management of acute and chronic pulpitis.

Understand the pathological changes involved in pulpitis.

Know how to recognize an alveolar abscess and be able to treat it.

Understand how infections can spread through the lymphous and the tissue spaces of the face.

Understand the management of infections about face.

▪ Key Concepts

Oral infections can be life threatening because of the following: ① a loss of the airway from swelling may result; ② infection may precipitate a systemic immune response. Early diagnosis and treatment is essential; it is unwise for oral and maxillofacial surgical departments not familiar with the day-to-day care of oral facial infections to monitor such patients. An understanding of the potential spaces in the oral and maxillofacial region is essential to ensure adequate drainage. Drainage and antibiotics remain the cornerstone of treatment.

▪ Introduction

Clinical symptoms and signs of infection may present within the orofacial region because of a localized infection, such as a bacterial abscess, or as part of the overall presentation of a systemic generalized infection. Infections within the orofacial region cause pain and debility and are a common source of lost working days. Occasionally they can be life threatening; in these cases, early and accurate diagnosis is required, followed by aggressive treatment and careful monitoring. Untreated, many initial acute infections will enter a chronic phase with persistence and further morbidity.

7.1 Pulpitis

Pulpitis inflammation of the pulp of a tooth and, in its acute form, is one of the most frequent emergencies facing the dentist. In the general there is a poor correlation between the patient's clinical symptoms and the findings when the pulp is examined histologically. The division of pulpitis based on predominantly on clinical symptoms. It should be remembered that pathological processes occurring in pulpitis may be completely asymptomatic.

7.2 Soft Tissue Infections of Face

7.2.1 Infection Sited a Tooth

Acute alveolar abscess: A common dental emergency facing the dentist is a patient with an acute alveolar abscess. There are a number of possible conditions that may lead to an abscess, including:

Periapical periodontitis.

Periodontal disease.

Periocoronitis.

Infection of cyst of the jaws.

Epidermoid cyst in the facial skin may become infected and be confused with infections of dental origin, according to their site, although a punctum marking the blocked keratinous outflow may be obvious.

7.2.1.1 Clinical features

There is severe pain that is not well localized, although the affected tooth is painful to touch when the abscess follows periapical periodontitis. The tooth is non-responsive to sensitivity tests and a history of trauma to a tooth may be implicated. More commonly, the tooth is carious on examination. Without treatment, the infection spreads through bone and periosteum producing a soft fluctuant swelling, which may be present in the buccal sulcus or occasionally in the palate. As soon as the abscess spreads out of bone and into soft tissues, there is a reduction in the pain experienced.

An abscess following periodontal disease is likely to result in a mobile tooth that is tender to percussion the tooth may remain responsive to sensitivity tests and any swelling is often nearer the gingival margin.

Trismus and cervical lymphadenopathy are signs of local spread of infection. Pyrexia and tachycardia are signs of systemic toxicity.

7.2.1.2 Management

The principle of treatment is to establish drainage of pus. In the case of a periapical abscess, this is may be a accomplished via the root canal after an air-rotor drill. This is does not require local anesthesia as the tooth is non-responsive to sensitivity tests, although it is important not to apply pressure to the tooth by cutting tooth is extracted to gain adequate drainage. This may be undertaken regional local anesthesia, with or without conscious sedation, or using general anesthesia.

7.2.2 Spread of Infection to Facial Tissues

7.2.2.1 Lymphatic spread of infection

The lymphatic system is frequently involved in infections and gives an indication as to the pattern of spread. Enlargement and tenderness of nodes, described as lymphadenitis, is common, although inflammation of the lymphatic vessels, described as lymphangitis, may occur and can be seen as thin red steaks through the skin.

7.2.2.2 Spread of infection through tissue spaces

In addition to spread through the lymphatic system, infection in the soft tissue of the face also spreads alone facial and muscle planes. These potential tissue spaces usually contain loose connective tissue and can be described anatomically.

7.2.2.3 Floor-of-mouth tissue spaces

The mylohyoid muscle divides the sublingual and submandibular spaces although they are continuous around its posterior free edge. The submental space is situated below the chin and between the anterior bellies of the digastric muscles. There are no restrictions on the spread of infection between the two submandibular spaces and the submental space; consequently, it can spread across the neck below the inferior border of the mandible.

7.2.2.4 Other tissues spaces of importance

Buccal spaces. These are located in the cheek on the lateral side of buccinators muscle. Submasseteric tissue spaces lie between the masseter muscle and the ramus of the mandible. The pterygomandibular space lies between the medical surface of the mandibular and the medial pterygoid muscle. The infratemporal space is the upper part of the pterygomandibular space and closely related to the upper molar teeth. The parotid space lies behind the ramus of the mandible and about the parotid gland.

Pharyngeal tissue spaces. Of these, the pharyngeal spaces are the most important in terms of spread of infection from the teeth and jaws. These spaces lie lateral to spaces, to where infection may spread. The retropharyngeal space, to where infection may spread. The retropharyngeal space lies behind the pharynx and in front of the prevertebral tonsil between the pillars of the fauces.

Hard palate area. There is no true tissue space in the hard palate because the mucosa is so tightly bound down to periosteum, but infection can strip away some of this and permit formation of an abscess.

7.2.2.5 Types of facial infection

(1) Maxillary infections

The spread of periapical infection may be predicted by the relationship of the buccinator muscle attachment to the teeth. Infection from the molar teeth usually spreads buccally or labially into the sulcus but may spread above the muscle into the superficial tissues of the cheek, where it can spread over a wide area with little to contain it. Infection frequently spreads to the palate from lateral incisors because of the palate inclination of the root. Occasionally, infection may also spread palatally from a palate root of a molar or premolar. The canine root is long and infection may spread superficially to the side of the nose rather than intra-orally.

(2) Mandibular infections

Periapical infection may similarly spread according to muscle attachments. Infection from incisors usually spreads labially into the sulcus but may spread to the chin between the two bellies of the mentalis muscle. Infection from the canine may spread into superficial tissues because the root is long. Premolars and molars show spread of infection into the buccal sulcus leading to the relation to the attachment of buccinators. Similarly, second mandibular molar teeth have more lingually placed root and may, therefore, result in either sublingual or submandibular spread depending on the relative position of the mylohyoid muscle (Figure 7-1).

(3) Cellulitis

Cellulitis is a spreading infection of connective tissue typical of streptococcal organisms. It spreads through the tissue spaces as described above and usually results from virulent and invasive organisms. The clinical features are those of a painful, diffuse, brawny swelling. The overlying skin is red, tense and shiny. There is usually an associated trismus, cervical lymphadenopathy, malaise and pyrexia.

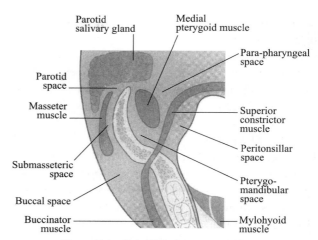

Figure 7-1 Potential tissue spaces about the posterior mandible

The swelling is the result of edema rather than pus and may be extensive when it involves lax tissue such as in the superficial mid-face about eyes. Cellulitis usually develops quickly, over the course of hours, and may follow an inadequately managed or ignored local dental infection.

If the infection spreads to involve the floor of the mouth and pharyngeal spaces, the airway can be compromised. Initially, the floor of the mouth will be raised and the patient will have difficult in swallowing saliva, this pools and may be observed running from the patient's mouth. This sign indicates the needs for urgent management. Cellulitis involving the tissue spaces on both sides of the floor of mouth is described as Ludwig's angina.

(4) Cavernous sinus thrombosis

Rarely infection in the tissues of the face may spread intracranially via the interconnecting venous system. This is more likely whit upper face via the facial vein to the cavernous sinus. While rare, cavernous sinus thrombosis is life threatening.

7.2.3 Management of the Infections about the Face

A clinical and radiographic examination of the mouth should be carried out to identify potential causes such as carious or partly erupted teeth or retained roots.

The patient may need to be admitted to hospital if they are unwell or there are signs of airway compromise. A differential white-cell count may indicate an increase in neutrophils. A blood glucose investigation may be carried out to exclude an underlying undiagnosed diabetes mellitus. Blood cultures should be performed if there is a spiking pyrexia or rigors. Intravenous antibiotics such as penicillin together with metronidazole should then be started, as well as fluids to rehydrate the patient, analgesics and antipyretic. Erythromycin or clindamycin may be appropriate if the patient is allergic to penicillin.

7.2.4 Drainage

Drainage should be established by opening or extracting the tooth or management as appropriate, such as for pericoronitis as described above. If there is an associated fluctuant swelling, then this may be incised and drained. This can be undertaken with ethyl chloride topical anesthesia, local anesthesia or general anesthesia as appropriate.

Drainage should not be delayed if the patient does not show signs of improvement. This may need to under general anesthesia if it is anticipated local anesthesia would be ineffective because of exquisite tenderness of the tooth or the extent of the swelling. The causative carious or impacted tooth or retained root should be removed at the same time. If trismus is a feature, intubation of the trachea will be difficult and the patient's air way will be at risk on induction of anesthesia. Such patients may need to undergo fibreoptic-assisted intubation while awake or sedated, prior to induction of anesthesia.

Drainage of tissue spaces may require extra-oral skin incision, blunt dissection to open abscess locules and insertion of a drain such as Yates to permit continued drainage for 24 – 48 hours. Pus is sent to microbiology laboratory for investigation of antibiotic sensitivity. When draining a cellulitis, little pus will be found, but tissue fluid will be released. In the case of Ludwig's angina, incisions are made bilaterally to drain the submandibular spaces via an extra-oral approach. The mortality of Ludwig's angina has reduced from 75% before advent of antibiotic use to 5%. A drain may be placed through the skin to protrude intra-orally. If the air way is at risk, the patient will remain intubated postoperatively and return to the intensive care unit for ventilation.

7.2.5 Chronic Infection

Acute infections may become chronic if treatment is inadequate. A persistent sinus may form, permitting intermittent discharge of pus. This may be intra-oral. The chronic infection may revert to an acute situation should the discharge be interrupted in any way.

■ Summary

The common clinical problems in dentistry are related to infections and inflammation. The most prevalent dental diseases, dental caries and the periodontal diseases, are not included here. However, the sequelae of these diseases are frequently infection inflammation of the bone. This chapter deals with these, along with other associated conditions of importance to dentist.

■ Questions

1. Orofacial infections are:
a. Common following contaminated facial laceration.
b. A common source of lost working days.
c. Usually of fungal or viral etiology when affecting the oral mucosa
d. Best managed by prescribing an antibiotic empirically rather than waiting for the results of a culture and sensitivity investigation
e. Commonly the result of the endogenous commensal organisms.

2. When would you use antibiotics to treat an infection of dental origin?

(**Xin Huang** 黄欣)

References

[1] Peter Ward Booth, Stephen A Schendel, Jarg-Erich Hausamen. Maxillofacial Surgery. 2nd ed. St. Louis, Missouri: Churchill Livingstone Elsevier, 2007: 1551-1571.
[2] Meurman JH, Hämäläinen P. Oral health and morbidity—implications of oral infections on the elderly. Gerodontology, 2006,23(1):3-16.
[3] Pussinen PJ, Mattila K. Periodontal infections and atherosclerosis: mere associations? Curr Opin Lipidol, 2004,15(5):583-588.
[4] Witherow H, Swinson BD, Amin M, et al. Management of oral and maxillofacial infection. Hosp Med, 2004,65(1):28-33.
[5] Heitmann C, Patzakis MJ, Tetsworth KD, et al. Musculoskeletal sepsis: principles of treatment. Instr Course Lect,2003,52:733-743.
[6] Fattahi TT, Lyu PE, Van Sickels JE. Management of acute suppurative parotitis. J Oral Maxillofac Surg,2002,60(4):446-448.

[7] Roberts G, Scully C, Shotts R. ABC of oral health. Dental emergencies. BMJ, 2000,321(7260):559-562.

[8] Flynn TR. The swollen face. Severe odontogenic infections. Emerg Med Clin North Am, 2000,18(3):481-519.

[9] Strachan DD, Williams FA, Bacon WJ. Diagnosis and treatment of pediatric maxillofacial infections. Gen Dent, 1998,46(2):180-182.

[10] Zeitoun IM, Dhanarajani PJ. Cervical cellulitis and mediastinitis caused by odontogenic infections: report of two cases and review of literature. J Oral Maxillofac Surg, 1995,53(2):203-208.

[11] McManners J, Samaranayake LP. Suppurative oral candidosis. Review of the literature and report of a case. Int J Oral Maxillofac Surg, 1990,19(5):257-259.

Chapter

Oral and Maxillofacial Injuries

▪ Objectives

Know how to carry a primary survey to identify and manage life threatening conditions.

Know how to access and document injuries.

Be aware of the particular requirements of a child patient.

Know the type of the dental injury that likely to occur.

Understand the management of such injuries.

Under the presentation and management of facial soft tissue injuries.

Know how to identify facial fractures clinically and radiologically.

Know the principles of management of different facial fractures.

Know the techniques use to fix the facial fractures.

▪ Key Concepts

In the emerging or third world countries, facial trauma is increasing rapidly mainly because of road traffic accidents, often involving pedestrians. Maxillofacial injures are common in patients with multiple trauma. These patients should be managed by a systemic initial care process, as outlined in advanced trauma life support (ATLS). Following primary stabilization, a thorough secondary survey is required by a specialist maxillofacial surgeon, with particular attention to head injures, uncontrolled facial/oral bleeding as well as abdominal and extremity trauma. Careful examination, correct diagnosis, careful treatment planning and accurate surgical technique will lead to optimal outcome for patients with maxillofacial injures.

▪ Introduction

Injures to the facial region are clinically highly significant for a number of reasons: ① the face provides anterior protection for the cranium; ② facial appearance is a highly significant factor in appearance, in most cultures; 3, the maxillofacial region is associated with a number of important functions of daily life, including sight, smell, eating, breathing, and talking; impairment in these functions severely affects the patient's quality of life. Maxillofacial injures occur in a variety of situations: road traffic accidents, inter-personal violence, or during sports. Patients with maxillofacial trauma demand good aesthetic and functional results, not only establishing a proper occlusion. With the methods and equipment currently available, especially the rigid internal fixation technique, maxillofacial surgeons can meet these demands.

8. 1   Assessment of the Injured Patient

Guidelines for the management of the injury trauma patent initially developed by the American college of surgeons have been widely adopted and disseminated through Advanced Trauma Life Support (ATLS) courses. These describe treatment priorities to achieve two aims: to save life and to restore function. A "primary survey" is carried out simultaneously to identify and to manage life threatening conditions and consists of the following (Figure 8-1):

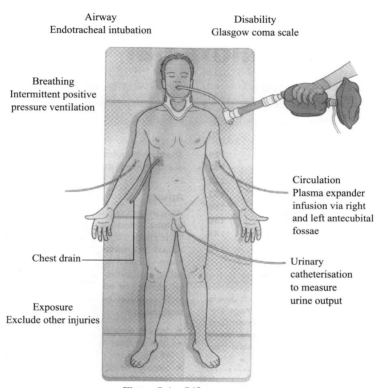

Airway
Endotracheal intubation

Disability
Glasgow coma scale

Breathing
Intermittent positive
pressure ventilation

Circulation
Plasma expander
infusion via right
and left antecubital
fossae

Chest drain

Urinary
catheterisation
to measure
urine output

Exposure
Exclude other injuries

Figure 8-1   Life support

Air way maintenance with cervical spine control.

Breathing and ventilation.

Circulation with control of hemorrhage.

Disability owing to neurological deficit.

Exposure and environmental control.

8. 1. 1   Airway

Airway management skills are necessary because the trauma patient will not be able to maintain his or her own airway if unconscious or if the airway is compromised by serious facial soft-tissue injury or facial fractures. However, airway skills are also important in other situations, such as when consciousness is altered by alcohol or other drugs, or when patients are treated with sedation and general anesthesia. It is important to understand:

How to recognize airway obstruction.

How to clear and maintain the airway with basic skills.

The role of advanced airway management including surgical managements.

Airway obstruction may be recognized by the "look, listen and fell" observations for breathing. Common causes of upper airway obstruction are the tongue and other soft tissues, blood, vomit, foreign body or edema. Obstruction may be partial or complete:

Silence suggest complete obstruction.

Gurgling suggest presence of liquid.

Snoring arises when pharynx is partially occluded by the tongue or soft palate.

Crowing is the sound of laryngeal spasm.

The jaw thrust is the method of choice for the trauma victim as this avoids extension of a potentially injured neck, and the nasopharyngeal airway should be avoid if a fracture of the maxilla is suspected as it may pass into the cranial fossa. Airway compromise resulting from facial injury will require the early involvement of the oral and the maxillofacial surgeon. Advanced airway management by way of endotracheal intubation is the "gold standard" of airway maintenance and protection but is only carried out in the trauma situation after cervical spine radiograph has excluded bone injury.

Surgical airway intervention may be indicated, as a life-saving procedure, if it is not possible to intubate the trachea. This may consist of a needle cricothyroidotomy, in which a large-calibre plastic cannula is inserted into the trachea through the cricothyroid membrane.

Alternatively, a surgical cricothyroidotomy may be undertaken with a transverse incision through the membrane to permit placement of a small endotracheal tube. These measures can provide up to 45 minutes of extra time in which to arrange undertaking emergency tracheostomy in theater environment. A transverse skin incision is made midway between the cricoid cartilage and the suprasternal notch followed by midline dissection of the infrahyoid muscles and division of the thyroid isthmus. Haemostasis is achieved and then the trachea is opened by cutting away part of the second and the third rings to create a circular opening so that a tracheostomy tube may be placed and secured (Figure 8-2).

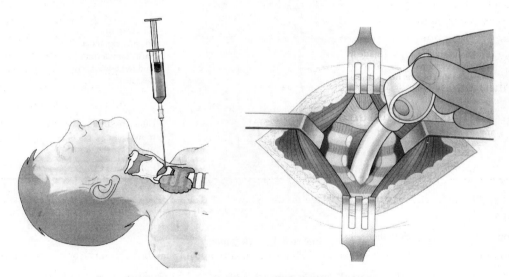

Figure 8-2   Cricothyroidotomy and tracheostomy

8.1.2   Breathing

Once an air way has been established, then the adequacy of ventilation must be assessed. Artificial ventilation must be commenced immediately when spontaneous ventilation is inadequate or absent. Serious chest injuries such as tension pneumothroax and cardiac tamponade will compromise spontaneous ventilation. Early diagnosis of these potentially life threatening conditions is essential so that they can be managed and permit adequate ventilation of patient.

8.1.3   Circulation

Hemorrhage should be controlled by pressure to bleeding wounds or by applying an artery forcep or ligature to a served artery as appropriate. Bleeding from a fractured maxilla will not be controlled unless it is manually repositioned, although this emergency is rare. If all local measures fail to control hemorrhage from the maxillofacial region then it may be necessary to consider ligation of the external carotid artery.

8. 1. 4 *Disability*
A rapid initial assessment of conscious state can be made using the APVU method: alert, responds to vocal stimulation, response to pain stimulation or unresponsive to all stimulation. Alternatively the Glasgow coma scale, which records the patient's motor, verbal and eye movements in response to simulation, may be used.

8. 1. 5 *Exposure and Environmental Control*
All of the victim's clothes are removed to permit full assessment and exclude other injuries, taking into account the environmental conditions and respecting the patients' dignity.

8. 1. 6 *Radiographic Examination*
Once immediate life-saving measure have been organized, essential radiography is undertaken. This is limited to cervical spine, chest and pelvis radiographs. The cervical spine is immobilized with a collar until any injury has been excluded.

8. 2 Dental Injuries

Dental injuries are common in children than adults. In children, they are frequently the result of falls and in adults they are commonly the consequence of sport without mouthguard protection. Increased overjet and incompetent lips are predisposing factors.

Definitions of a few basic terms are useful:

Concussion. A traumatic event leads to damage to the periodontium without loosening or displacement of the tooth.

Subluxation. Damage to the periodontium leads to loosening of the tooth without over displacement.

Luxation. This is the term given to dislocation of the tooth within socket, leading to loosening and some degree of displacement. Luxation can be intrusive, extrusive or lateral in direction.

Avulsion. The tooth is completely displaced from its socket.

Table 8-1 gives the management for injures to primary and permanent tooth. Reassurance and analgesia are especially important to children. Patients will require regular review to assess development of late sequelae.

If there has been any loss of consciousness at the time of injuries and a tooth or part of a tooth has been lost, then a chest radiography should be arranged to confirm that this has not been inhaled.

Splints can be directly constructed in the mouth of the patient or indirectly constructed on a model in a laboratory. Direct splints may be made from foil in adapted to over the teeth and cemented with zinc oxide eugenol or better with composite that is attached to the teeth over a wire using an acid-etch technique.

Table 8-1 Management of tooth injuries

Injury	Management
Primary tooth	
Concussion	Soft diet
Crown fracture	Smooth or restore (when root canal treatment may be necessary) or extract depending on extent
Root fracture	Soft diet or extract if cause crown mobility
Luxation	Soft diet
Intrusion	Leave to erupt (when may be require later pulp treatment) or extract if radiography suggests underlying permanent follicle involved.
Avulsion	Do not re-implant
Permanent tooth	
Concussion	Soft diet
Enamel fracture	Smooth or restore
Fracture involving dentine	Protect dentine and restore

Continue

Injury	Management
Fracture involving pulp	Pulp cap (<1 mm exposure) or pulpotomy (>1 mm exposure) when the apex is open; pulp cap (if immediate presentation) or pulpectomy (if later presentation) when apex is closed.
Root fracture	Splint two weeks if mobile Apical or middle third: root treat to fracture line Coronal third: extract coronal part of tooth and restore root after gingivectomy or orthodontic extrusion Vertical: extract
Luxation	Reposition tooth manually under local anesthesia and splint (2 weeks) followed by root treatment as necessary
Intrusion	Leave to erupt when apex is open or use orthodontic extrusion if apex closed, followed by root treatment as necessary
Extrusion	Reposition tooth manually under local anesthesia and splint (2 weeks) followed by root treatment as necessary
Avulsion	Less than 1 hour since avulsion; irrigate with saline and replant (tooth should have been stored in saliva milk or preferably); compress the socket; splint (for approximately 7 days) and prescribe antibiotics and chlorhexidine, followed by root treatment as necessary Tooth avulsed for more than 30 minutes or apex closed; root treat with calcium hydroxide

8.3 **Facial Soft Tissue Injuries**

8.3.1   *Etiology*
Soft tissue injury may result from interpersonal violence, road traffic accident. Weapons may not be involved. Facial injury may also result from burns either as an isolated injury or in association with burns of the trunk or other part of body.

8.3.2   *Clinical Presentation*
Lacerations and wounds may involve anatomical structures such as the facial nerve, resulting in facial paralyze, the parotid salivary gland duct, resulting in a salivary fistula, or arteries, resulting in a significant blood loss. They may be "clean" or obviously contaminated. Burns are described according to their depth and extent. They may be superficial (first-degree burn), partial thickness (second-degree burn) or full thickness (third-degree burn). The "rule of nines" may be use to describe the total body surface area affected by burn: 9% for each arm the head, 18% for each leg, front and back of trunk and 1% for the external genitalia. The rule is modified for children who have a relatively larger head and face. The estimation is important for calculating fluid replacement.

8.3.3   *Radiology*
Radiographs of the soft tissue may be necessary to locate glass or other foreign body in a wound or to exclude an underlying bony injury. Soft tissue radiographs are taken with reduced exposure to avoid "burn-out" of low-density debris, and using intra-oral films wherever for greatest detail.

8.3.4   *Surgical Management of Lacerations*
Small, straightforward lacerations may be managed by accident and emergency physicians or senior nurses. Lacerations involving the vermilion border of the lip, intra-oral lacerations and gunshot wounds will be referred on to an oral and maxillofacial surgeon. General dentists may undertake management of intra-oral lacerations in primary care situation.

Small lacerations usually be sutured under local anesthesia is indicated. Thorough cleaning is necessary before wound closure. Skin lacerations are closed with fine non-absorbable material such as polyglactin placed deep if necessary and then the overlying skin closed with fine non-absorbable material such as 6/0 prolene or ethilon. Intra-oral wounds may be closed with vicryl or silk. It is important when repairing a lip laceration which involves the vermilion border that it is accurately lined up to avoid an ugly step on healing.

Alternate skin sutures should ideally be removed at 4 days and the remaining sutures at 5 days to minimize scarring while maintaining wound support.

8.4 Facial Fractures

8.4.1 Clinical Presentation

8.4.1.1 Mandible

(1) Pain and swelling.

(2) Deranged occlusion.

(3) Paraesthesia in distribution area of inferior alveolar nerve.

(4) Floor-of-mouth hematoma.

8.4.1.2 Zygoma

(1) Clinical flattening of the cheek bone prominence.

(2) Paraesthesia in distribution area of infra-orbital nerve.

(3) Diplopia, restricted eye movement, subconjunctival hemorrhage.

(4) Limited lateral excursions of mandibular movements.

(5) Palpable step in infra-orbital bony margin.

8.4.1.3 Orbit

Diplopia, restricted eye movement, subconjunctival hemorrhage.

8.4.1.4 Maxilla

(1) Maxilla mobile.

(2) Deranged occlusion.

(3) Gross swelling if high-level fracture.

(4) Bilateral circumorbital bruising.

(5) Subconjunctival hemorrhage.

(6) Cerebrospinal fluid leaking from nose (rhinorrhea) or ear.

8.4.2 Principles of Facial Fracture Management

Good bony healing of fractures requires close apposition of the fragments and immobility for a period of about 6 weeks. This period may be shorter in children and longer in elderly patients. Mobility of the fracture site will lead to fibrous union. The principles of fracture management are, therefore, those of reduction and fixation.

There many different techniques for fixation of facial fractures and these may be described as rigid, semi-rigid or non-rigid. The fracture site may be surgically opened and fixation such as plates applied. There has been a move in the developed world towards greater use of direct fixation of fractures rather than indirect, but the latter does still have particular indications.

8.4.3 Dento-alveolar Fractures

Fractures of the tooth-bearing part of the mandible or maxilla are reduced and then immobilized by one of the many methods. All techniques involving fixing the teeth involved in the fracture to adjacent teeth, and this may be achieved by means of writing arch bars, acid-etch-retained composite splinting, orthodontic banding or cement-retained acrylic splints. Splinting is required for a minimum of 4 weeks.

8.4.4 Mandibular Fractures

Fractures are classified according to their site: dento-alveolar, symphyseal, parasymphyseal, body, angle, ramus, coronoid and condyle (Figure 8-3). They may be compound, involving the mouth or skin, or may be simple or comminuted. It is more unusual to describe fractures as favorable or unfavorable according to whether the resists the pull of attached muscles. The standard treatment is open reduction and internal fixation (ORIF) with miniplates. This approach has revolutionized the managment of mandibular fractures and also other facial fractures. A fractures of mandible un a dentate patient may typically be reduced and fixed with intermaxillary fixation (IMF) achieve by placement of arch bars.

If there is partly erupted or erupted tooth in the line of fracture, one should consider whether it ought to be removed or avoid predisposing to later infection of the fracture site or whether it could remain. Most surgeons would leave the tooth in situ unless it is fractured, grossly carious or has periapical pathology.

Fractures of the condyle not interfering with the occlusion are frequently managed conservatively, that is with soft diet and regular review. A 2-week period of IMF rather than ORF is a common treatment choice if the occlusion is deranged.

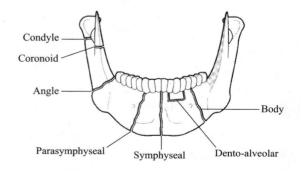

Condyle

Coronoid

Angle

Body

Parasymphyseal   Symphyseal   Dento-alveolar

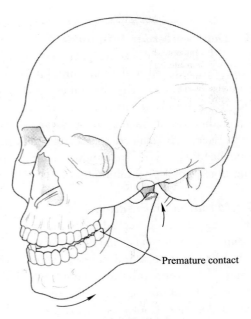

Figure 8-3   Mandibular fractures

8.4.5   Zygoma Fractures

Zygoma fractures are most commonly reduced by elevation via a Gillies' temporal approach. A Rowe's elevator is placed beneath the deep temporal fascia, slid under the zygoma and lifted without levering on the temporal bone. Alternative methods include an intra-oral approach and direct lifting of zygoma with a hook placed through the skin of the check. The zygoma may or may not net fixation depending on its stability. When needed titanium miniplates may be placed at the zygomatic-frontal, infra-orbital and buttress regions as necessary.

8.4.6   Orbital Fractures

Fractures of the zygomatic complex will necessary involve the orbit, but it is also possible to sustain an isolated fracture of the orbit. This is may tether the inferior rectus muscle, causing diplopia, or be large enough to permit herniation of orbital fat and muscle into maxillary antrum. Such a "blow-out" may be repaired with "silastic" or titanium mesh materials or bone taken from another site, for example iliac crest of the hip or the cranium.

8.4.7   Maxillary Fractures

Fractures of the maxilla are classified as Le Fort I, II, III (Figure 8-4). Le Fort I is the lowest level of fracture, in which the tooth-bearing part of the maxilla is detached, Le Fort II or a pyramidal fracture of maxilla involves the nasal bones and infra-orbital rims, while Le Fort III involves the nasal bones and zygomatic-frontal sutures and the whole of the maxilla is detached from the base of the skull. After reduction of the fracture, fixation may be achieved by a variety of means, including directly applied plates and indirect fixation such as a external frame made of stainless steel pins, rods and universal joints fixing the maxilla to the cranium. Intermaxillary fixation may also be required.

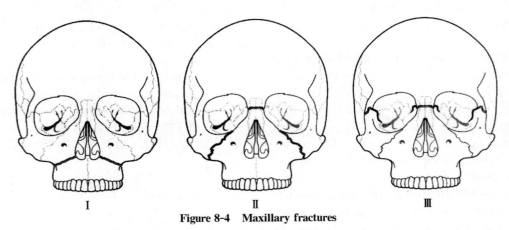

I   II   III

Figure 8-4   Maxillary fractures

■ Summary

This chapter concentrates on injuries to the face. It covers the primary survey produce to identify and manage life threatening injuries and the subsequent assessment and care of injuries that occur to teeth, soft tissue and bones of the face. The techniques available for fixing facial fractures are described.

■ Questions

1. Fractures involving the orbit:
a. May increase the volume of the orbit
b. Are described either as "blow-out" or as "blow-in" fractures
c. May be complicated by blindness
d. Always require surgical repair
e. May cause subconjunctival hemorrhage
2. Fractures of maxilla:
a. Are less frequent if seat belts are worn
b. May cause limited opening of the mandible
c. May be suspected if there is intra-oral bruising
d. May result in severe hemorrhage
e. Can result from less force than required to facture the mandible
3. What surgical techniques are available for the management of fractures to the mandible?
4. What are some of the complications that may arise during mandibular fracture management?
5. How many dento-alveolar fractures should be managed?
6. Describe the management of a laceration to the tongue.

(Xin Huang　黄欣)

References

[1] Peter Ward Booth, Stephen A Schendel, Jarg-Erich Hausamen. Maxillofacial Surgery. 2nd ed. St. Louis, Missouri: Churchill Livingstone Elsevier, 2007: 13-15.
[2] Delantoni A, Antoniades I. The iatrogenic fracture of the coronoid process of the mandible. A review of the literature and case presentation. Cranio, 2010,28(3):200-204.
[3] Sharif MO, Fedorowicz Z, Drews P, et al. Interventions for the treatment of fractures of the mandibular condyle. Cochrane Database Syst Rev, 2010,14(4):CD006538.
[4] Pedroletti F, Johnson BS, McCain JP. Endoscopic techniques in oral and maxillofacial surgery. Oral Maxillofac Surg Clin North Am, 2010, 22(1):169-182.
[5] Dupanovic M, Fox H, Kovac A. Management of the airway in multitrauma. Curr Opin Anaesthesiol, 2010, 23(2):276-282.
[6] Bourguignon C, Sigurdsson A. Preventive strategies for traumatic dental injuries. Dent Clin North Am, 2009,53(4):729-749, vii.
[7] Stefanopoulos PK, Tarantzopoulou AD. Management of facial bite wounds. Dent Clin North Am, 2009, 53(4):691-705.
[8] Perry M. Maxillofacial trauma—developments, innovations and controversies. Injury, 2009, 40(12):1252-1259.
[9] Bell RB. Management of frontal sinus fractures. Oral Maxillofac Surg Clin North Am, 2009, 21(2):227-242.
[10] Kontio R, Lindqvist C. Management of orbital fractures. Oral Maxillofac Surg Clin North Am, 2009, 21(2):209-220, vi.
[11] Myall RW. Management of mandibular fractures in children. Oral Maxillofac Surg Clin North Am, 2009, 21(2):197-201, vi.
[12] Laskin DM. Management of condylar process fractures. Oral Maxillofac Surg Clin North Am, 2009, 21(2):193-196, v-vi.
[13] Ellis E. Management of fractures through the angle of the mandible. Oral Maxillofac Surg Clin North Am, 2009, 21(2):163-174.
[14] Valiati R, Ibrahim D, Abreu ME, et al. The treatment of condylar fractures: to open or not to open? A critical review of this controversy. Int J Med Sci, 2008, 5(6):313-318.
[15] Wang D, Levin LS. Composite tissue transfer in upper extremity trauma. Injury, 2008, 39 (Suppl 3):S90-96.
[16] Nussbaum ML, Laskin DM, Best AM. Closed versus open reduction of mandibular condylar fractures in adults: a meta-analysis. J Oral Maxillofac Surg, 2008, 66(6):1087-1092.
[17] Sauerbier S, Schön R, Otten JE, et al. The development of plate osteosynthesis for the treatment of fractures of the mandibular body—a literature review. J Craniomaxillofac Surg, 2008, 36(5):251-259.
[18] Perry M, Morris C. Advanced trauma life support (ATLS) and facial trauma: can one size fit all? Part 2: ATLS, maxillofacial injuries and airway management dilemmas. Int J Oral Maxillofac Surg, 2008, 37(4):309-320.
[19] Perry M. Advanced trauma life support (ATLS) and facial trauma: can one size fit all? Part 1: dilemmas in the management of the multiply injured patient with coexisting facial injuries. Int J Oral Maxillofac Surg, 2008, 37(3):209-214.
[20] Perry M, O'Hare J, Porter G. Advanced trauma life support (ATLS) and facial trauma: can one size fit all? Part 3: Hypovolaemia and facial injuries in the multiply injured patient. Int J Oral Maxillofac Surg, 2008, 37(5):405-414.
[21] Perry M, Moutray T. Advanced trauma life support (ATLS) and facial trauma: can one size fit all? Part 4: 'can the patient see?' Timely diagnosis, dilemmas and pitfalls in the multiply injured, poorly responsive/unresponsive patient. Int J Oral Maxillofac Surg, 2008, 37(6):505-514.
[22] Combes JG, Gibbons AJ. Oral and maxillofacial surgery. J R Army Med Corps, 2007, 153(3):205-209.
[23] Hermund NU, Hillerup S, Kofod T, et al. Effect of ear-

ly or delayed treatment upon healing of mandibular fractures: a systematic literature review. Dent Traumatol, 2008, 24(1):22-26.

[24] Andrade MG, Weissman R, Oliveira MG, et al. Tooth displacement and root dilaceration after trauma to primary predecessor: an evaluation by computed tomography.

Dent Traumatol, 2007, 23(6):364-367.

[25] Ceallaigh PO, Ekanaykaee K, Beirne CJ, et al. Diagnosis and management of common maxillofacial injuries in the emergency department. Part 5: Dentoalveolar injuries. Emerg Med J, 2007, 24(6):429-430.

Chapter 9

Temporomandibular Disorders

- **Objectives**

The objective is to introduce the pathogenesis of the temporomandibular disorders.

- **Key concepts**

Temporomandibular disorders, occlusion, intracapsular disorders

- **Introduction**

Temporomandibular disorders include occluso-muscle disorders and intracapsular disorders of TMJ.

9.1 Making Sense of Terminology

Temporomandibular disorder (TMD) is any disorder that affects or is affected by deformity, disease, misalignment, or dysfunction of the temporomandibular articulation and/or masticatory muscles.

In etiologic studies, and in much of dental education, has been in the context of a single, multifactorial syndrome that includes disorders that are unrelated to the temporomandibular articulation and are often even unrelated to any masticatory system consideration. Even when TMD is shown to occur in different forms, or when variations of symptoms are categorized, such categorizations have typically been clustered into a syndrome rather than as distinctly different and specific types of disorders with different etiologies requiring specifically directed treatment.

Occlusal disharmony that affects the position of the TMJs, and disorders of the masticatory musculature are also included as specific types of TMDs. Never use the term TMD without specific classification of the exact type of disorder being discussed, and the structures that are affected.

9.2 Occluso-muscle Disorders

9.2.1 Principle

Most temporomandibular disorder (TMD) pain is not temporomandibular joint (TMJ) pain. Most TMD pain is masticatory muscle pain triggered by deflective occlusal interferences.

Occluso-muscle disorder: discomfort or dysfunction resulting from hyperactive, incoordinated muscle function that is triggered by deflective occlusal interferences to physiologic jaw movements and noxious habits.

It is significant that the most common and most correctable cause of orofacial pain is not defined in dental glossaries. Occluso-muscle disorders are, without doubt, the most prevalent cause of orofacial pain. Even in tertiary pain patients, occluso-muscle pain is the most common finding. Occluso-muscle pain is also the most misunderstood and the most ignored of all the masticatory system disorders.

9.2.2 Diagnosing Occluso-muscle Pain

Learning to separate occluso-muscle pain from a TMD is an essential part of differentiating types of pain and can cause diverse side effects such as headaches and neck aches. It is important to examine each aspect of the pain in search of its cause.

Examine range of motion:

Two factors limit normal range of motion (ROM):

(1) Muscle hypercontraction

(2) Joint immobility due to an intracapsular disorder

Observer for smooth, symmetrical, nonlimited movement of wide, left, right, and protrusive openings.

General normals: wide   40 – 50 mm
lateral   7 – 15 mm
protrusive   7 – 15 mm

What muscle palpation tells us:

The standard screening exam for TMDs includes palpation of the masticatory muscles. Muscle tenderness can almost always be related to hyperactivity of the muscle as a result of overworked when it is required to constantly hold the jaw in an avoidance pattern during closure to maximum intercuspation. Analysis of which muscles are sore should be related to the direction of mandibular displacement at tooth contact. If the deflective tooth incline re-lates to the muscles that are tender to palpation, it is an indication of occluso-muscle pain.

9.2.3 Testing

Lateral pterygoid muscle: Palpation of the lateral pterygoid muscle is not practical, but it can be tested effectively to see if it is a source of pain.

Hyoid area: The digastric and the hyoid muscles are often involved when deflective occlusal interferences cause the mandible to be posture forward to avoid the interferences.

Sternocleidomastoid (SCM) muscle: If this muscle is tender to palpation, evaluate collateral effects from head posture and/or cervical misalignments. Consider referral to a physical therapist for adjunctive evaluation. Be aware that occlusal disharmony is not the only cause for head and neck muscle problems.

Occipital area: Occipital headaches are commonly associated with occlusal interferences. If tender, look for occlusal interferences to centric relation or excursions. Recognize that this problem may result in combination with head posture and cervical misalignments, or it may be unrelated to occlusal factors. Consider referral to a physical therapist for adjunctive therapy.

Trapezius muscle: In spite of claims that a form of TMD includes shoulder and back pain, clinical experience indicates that while some pain in this area does disappear when the occlusion is corrected, the result is probably more related to the improvement of head posture that is common when occlusal disharmony is corrected. Cervical misalignment must always be a consideration. Consider referral to a physical therapist.

Confirmative diagnosis: The reason occluso-muscle pain should never be missed as a diagnosis because the diagnosis can be confirmed by two simple tests.

9.3 Intracapsular Disorders of the TMJ

Principle

The condition of the intracapsular structure of the temporomandibular joints (TMJs) affects the position of the TMJs. Consequently it affects the jaw-to-jaw occlusal relationship.

9.3.1 Intracapsular Pain

Many different types of disorders can affect the tissues within the capsule of the TMJ. Deformation of intracapsular structures can produce a variety of different pain symptoms depending on which tissues are affected, the degree and type of damage, variations in compressive or tensive forces applied, and the response to varying levels of pain.

9.3.2 The Healthy Joint
Description

The healthy TMJ is aligned in the center of its disk. Both the condyle and eminence are convex and are covered with intact fibrocartilage over a dense cortical bone layer. The disk is firmly attached to the lateral and medial poles of the condyle. The retrodiscal tissues that compose the bilaminar posterior attachment of the disk are intact, and the superior strata exert an elastic pull oil the disk.

Treatment

Occlusal correction is indicated to eliminate all interferences to centric relation and to correct excursive pathways. The manipulation into centric relation must be verified to ensure correct disk alignment. The treatment method of choice is selected after analysis of the mounted casts. If interim treatment is needed for some purpose, a full occlusal bite plane can be constructed as a temporary procedure. If a bite plane is used, it should be meticulously adjusted to centric relation, and the anterior guidance on the bite plane should disclude tile posterior teeth in all excursions.

9.3.3 Lateral Pole Disk Displacement

Now the reciprocal click is introduced. It results from a reducible displacement of the disk in front of the lateral pole of the condyle.

Description

At this stage of progression, the lateral discal ligament and the posterior condylar attachment of the disk have been stretched or torn sufficiently to allow the lateral half of the posterior band of the disk to displace completely in front of the lateral pole of the condyle. The lateral pole of the condyle now rests against the vascular, innervated tissue behind the disk. The medial pole is still positioned in its concavity between the anterior and posterior bands of the disk, but from that point laterally the disk has been deranged anteromedially.

Treatment

If prolonged use of a bite plane is desired, it should include the full occlusion harmonized to a verified centric relation. Do not use any segmental bite plane for more than a few days. Once the diag-

nosis is confirmed by the anterior bite plane. It is logical to proceed with your selected occlusal treatment. Finalization of the occlusion may not be possible, however, until some remodeling occurs in the deformed disk. If the occlusion is to be restored, equilibration should be done first until a point of stability is reached. This can be done directly or on a superior repositioning splint.

9.3.4 Lateral Pole Closed Lock

At this stage, the click goes away, but it is not because the joint healed itself. It is because tile problem progressed. The lateral part of the posterior band thickens and locks in front of the lateral pole of the condyle.

Description

The disk is rotated medioanteriorly so that the medial pole of the condyle is still between the anterior an posterior bands of the disk but the posterior band crosses over the condyle diagonally, putting tile lateral part of the posterior band in front of the condyle.

Treatment

Even though considerable changes have taken place in the joint, the deformation through this stage is transient. Some derangement of fibers may occur in the disk, but it is still elastic enough to revert to its initial fiber pattern lf the load is redirected through the central beating area. In treating this stage of derangement, special care must be taken to ensure that the entire disk has been recaptured and that it stays recaptured during function. Unless the joint is tested carefully with very firm bilateral pressure, it is easy to be misled about the alignment of the disk because the medial pole can still accept most of the load without discomfort. Doppler auscultation of the TMJ is excellent for verifying that the disk has been completely recaptured. This is because crepitus will be eliminated, or barely audible crepitation will be noticed that probably results from seine residual changes in the surface of the disk.

9.3.5 Complete Anterior Disk Displacement

At this stage, the problem gets more serious. The disk is completely displaced forward of the condyle.

9.3.5.1 Description

The discal ligaments to the lateral half of the disk have now been torn or stretched far enough to allow severe medioanterior displacement of the disk, As this occurs, more and more of the posterior band of tile disk is progressively forced in front of the condyle until the entire posterior band has become anteriorly displaced. The condyle is now loaded entirely on the vascular, innervated retrodiscal tissues. In protrusive movements of the condyle, there is now a progressive tendency to force the disk ahead of the condyle while compressively loading the entire width of the posterior attachments to the disk.

Scapino has shown that the posterior attachments to the disk may respond to this forward thrust by moving the condylar attachment of the posterior ligament up the posterior surface of the condyle through bony remodeling at the attachment site. A response to excessive traction can occur either at the condylar attachment of the posterior ligament or at the temporal bone attachment of the superior strata of elastic fibers. The apparent reason for moving the anchorage of the elastic fibers forward rather than just allowing them to stretch is probably related to the common finding of fibrosis in the elastic fibers of deranged disks. The fibrosis would remarkably reduce the elasticity of the posterior attachment and thus increase the tension on the site of the attachment at the temporal bone.

The forward migration of the temporal attachment does not seem to require bony remodeling as is seen in the forward repositioning of the inelastic collagen fibers that attach the disk to the condyle. This forward attachment of the elastic fibers might also occur as a result of fibrous ankylosis initiated by intracapsular bleeding. Piper reports a fairly common occurrence of such ankylosis or adhesion in the retrodiscal tissues that have been damaged by direct loading from the condyle when the disk is anteriorly displaced.

9.3.5.2 Variations of disk displacements

There are many variations of complete disk displacement. In the early stages, the medial pole is usually reducible even if the lateral pole is not, because at the medial pole the anterior and posterior raised bands are often still intact and separated long after the lateral part of the disk has become irreducibly altered. The separation of the two bands provides a concave bearing area for the medial pole of the condyle just as long and only as long as the condyle can get past the posterior band and into the seating position between the two raised bands. In time, however, the breakdown of the posterior ligament progressively weakens the medial attachment of the disk, just as it has occurred at the lateral

pole. So eventually the disk displacement becomes irreducible at the medial pole also. The resultant closed lock of tile entire disk is subject to the same progressive changes that have been described for the lateral pole. All of the changes that now occur are dependent on time intensity, and direction of the load applied through the condyle, tempered by the response of host resistance. It is, simply stated, a matter of adaptive response. The adaptive process can be destructive, or it can be beneficial.

The most common disk deformities that occur with complete displacement are as follows:

(1) The disk is misshapened but is recapturable by both medial and lateral poles.

(2) The disk may be folded at the lateral portion but not at the medial bearing area.

(3) The disk is folded through its full width, so the central bearing area is narrowed or is obliterated completely.

(4) The disk has become remodeled so that it is potentially recapturable at the medial pole only.

(5) The disk is nonreducible, and the entire bearing area between the anterior and posterior bands has been obliterated by nonreversible remodeling changes.

9.3.5.3 Signs and symptoms

The principal early symptom in complete anterior displacements is pain in the joint region combined with varying degrees of muscle pain. The patient may be unable to precisely locate the focus of pain because it so often is commingled. At the early stages, the loaded rotrodiscal tissues are still vascular and richly innervated, so compression can cause severe pain. As compressive changes occur in the tissues, the normal pattern of vascular retrodiscal tissues may be replaced by a more compact mass of fibers that are almost devoid of the small vessels that were originally present. As the vessels disappear from the bearing area, the pain diminishes. If the adaptive remodeling response is successful, a new avascular bearing pad of fibers that provides a pain-free extension to the disk may be formed. This is often an acceptable substitute for the original correctly aligned disk. From this potential response to displacement, one can see that the symptom of pain can vary from extreme pain to no pain, depending on how the compressed tissues adapt.

Since pain is the most important symptom to consider in determining treatment, it should be evaluated carefully to determine its source. In a large number of patients with complete disk displacements, I have observed the pain almost entirely attributable to muscle incoordination, with little or none in the joint itself. Such patients generally respond well to occlusal therapy.

The principal sign associated with complete disk displacement is clicking. As long as the disk displacement is reducible, a click will be observed on opening as the condyle clicks onto the disk, followed by a reciprocal click upon closing as the condyle slips back off the disk.

When the elastic fibers lose their ability to overcome the forward push of the motive condyle against the disk, the clicks disappear, indicating a closed lock. From that point on, the potential for degenerative joint disease increases.

9. 3. 5. 4   Methods of diagnosis

(1) History.

(2) Clinical observations

On opening, the jaw will normally deviate toward the side of the displacement, sometimes very sharply. If the displacement is reducible, the reducing condyle may suddenly, jump forward, bringing the mandible back to a more centered relationship after reduction. If it is nonreducing, the mandible may stay deviated upon opening.

It is difficult or impossible to move the jaw laterally away from the displaced side, but it moves easily toward the displaced side. If reduction occurs immediately upon opening, the posterior attachments to the disk are still reasonably intact.

If reduction does not occur before the condyle has translated forward about 3mm (about two finger widths of opening), the posterior attachment may be damaged too badly to recapture the disk and have it stay recaptured during function.

(3) Manipulative testing

If the condyle is loaded with upward pressure against vascular innervated tissue, there will be some response of tenderness or tension. With newly displaced disks, pressure may cause sharp pain. The discomfort must be distinguished from that caused by applied tension against the contracted lateral pterygoid muscle or from pathosis, but any sign of discomfort should alert us to the possibility of disk displacement. Use of other diagnostic tests may be necessary to distinguish between the other possibilities of pathosis, or muscle bracing.

If a disk displacement is confirmed but loading of the joint does not cause discomfort, it is an indi-

cation that adaptive remodeling may have altered the retrodiscal tissues to form a new bearing pad extension of the displaced disk. Even though the disk may be displaced, the new alignment may be acceptable if it permits medial-pole bracing of the condyle. The same may be true in some bone-to-bone relationships if the articulating surfaces of the condyle and eminence have remodeled to hard eburnated surfaced.

Manipulative loading of the joints is an extremely valuable test to determine whether an acceptable level of comfort can be achieved with the present conditions.

(4) Palpation

Finger pressure through the skin depression behind the condyle when the jaw is open will usually provoke tenderness in varying degrees depending on the condition of the posterior attachment. Palpation of masticatory muscles is almost certain to cause a tenderness response in the incoordinated muscles that are involved in the jaw displacement.

(5) Auscultation

Doppler auscultation of the TMJ is all almost foolproof method for determining whether or not the condyle is on the disk. It is also very reliable for determining the precise point of recapture and displacement when the disk is reducible because the reciprocal clicks are audible even when they cannot be heard through a stethoscope.

The character of the amplified crepitus sounds is also diagnostic: the coarser the crepitus, the more there is breakdown of the posterior ligament. Chirping sounds indicate perforation of the ligament. If the chirping is mixed with very coarse crepitus, there is a probability that the posterior ligament has been severely damaged or lost and there is a bone-to-bone articulation.

Ankylosis of the disk would produce opening and closing clicks at the same protrusive position of the condyle. If the disk is not ankylosed but is still reducible, the opening click usually occurs at a more open relationship than the closing click. If the disk is not recapturable, crepitus will be heard for all jaw movements and there will be no click.

(6) Radiographic findings

If the disk is completely displaced, lateral transcranial radiographs usually show the condyle distal to a centralized position in the fossa. The space above the condyle is often diminished also, but the diagnosis cannot be based solely on transcranial radiographs because variations in condyle-fossa contour can cause an appearance of displacement when one does not exist. Variations in beam angulation can also distort the apparent condyle position, and so transcranial radiographs should always be used in combination with other diagnostic tests. Nevertheless transcranial radiographs have great value in many instances, often disclosing important information about the condition of the condyle or eminence such as remodeling changes at the bony surfaces, degenerative joint disease, or other forms of pathosis.

(7) Arthrography

Although arthrography is rarely used today because of the availability of noninvasive MRI, we learned much about how the disk responds in many different deformative conditions from early studies. Combining arthrography with fluoroscopy, we were able to see the action of the disk during function (Figures 9-1 and 9-2). Through **differential arthrography**, a method developed by Mark Piper, we were able to observe the effect of muscle incoordination on disk alignment. While observing the position of nonreducible disks via the fluoroscope, then anesthetizing the motor in nervation to the superior lateral pterygoid muscle, it became evident that muscle contraction played a dominant role in disk displacement. In some TMJs the disk spontaneously reduced when the muscle was anesthetized.

(8) Magnetic resonance imaging

Today the unquestioned gold standard for diagnosis of disk derangements is MRI. The consequences of complete disk displacement are too varied to trust to guessing what the condition or position of the disk is. Because of the work of Schellhas, precise procedures for imaging the TMJs make it possible to see the exact position and condition of the disk on both the medial and lateral poles of the condyle. In addition to assessing soft tissues. MRI shows bone marrow changes, disk morphology, mobility, and Joint effusion.

MRI is typically reserved for complete disk derangements or when unexplainable pain or dysfunction of the TMJs is present that does not respond to treatment. there is a simple rule to follow in regard to all TMJ problems: the joint cannot comfortably accept loading, find out why. If routine diagnostic procedures do not reveal the cause of the pain or dysfunction, MRI is recommended. It would he an unwise decision to proceed with extensive occlusal therapy, orthodontics, or restorative treatment in the presence of au undiagnosed TMD.

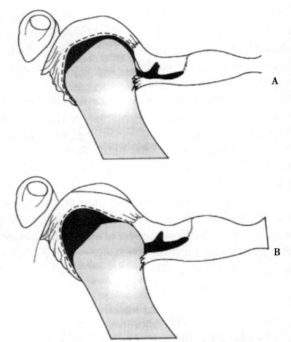

Figure 9-1   Early arthrographic studies combined with fluoroscopy show the action of a displaced disk during function

A. The dye pattern in retruded position. Notice that the dye extends well forward of the condyle in the inferior joint space and outlines the underside of the disk. The posterior band has been pushed forward, nearly obliterating the normal seating area for the condyle. In B, the disk has been shoved ahead of the protruding condyle without reduction. Diagnosis: nonreducible disk derangement. Disk is not bound down and is most likely reparable. In some joints. anesthetizing the superior lateral pterygoid motor-innervation caused the disk to spontaneously reduce

(9) Computed tomography

CT is very useful for assessing abnormalities of bone such as ankylosis, dysplasias, growth abnormalities, fractures, and osseous tumors. With the manufacture of head/neck CT scanners, precise analysis of the condyle position, contour, and bone surfaces is possible. Structural analysis of the temporomandibular articulation can, today, be as complete as is necessary to arrive at an accurate diagnosis.

New imaging technology offers unparalleled opportunities to examine all of the bony structures in masticatory system. The NewTom CT scanner facilitates thin 1mm slices from any direction through the TMJ and other structures. The combination of CT and MRI has opened the door to much better understanding of disorders in both hard and soft tissues of the masticatory system. Today it is almost impossible for a structural disorder of the TMJs to hide from a knowledgeable clinician.

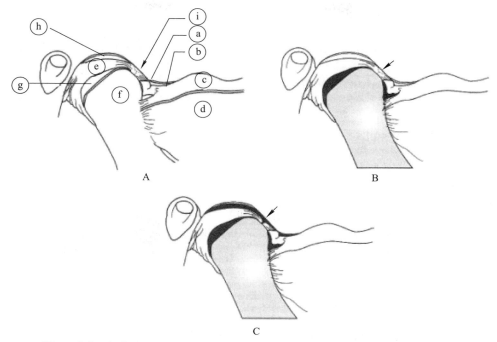

Figure 9-2 Arthrogram pattern when there is a perforation in the retrodiscal tissues
Notice how dye leaks through from the inferior joint space into the superior joint space. In this illustration, the disk is folded in front of the protrudent condyle. **A.** Orientation of tissues; posterior band of disk. a: anterior band of disk, b: superior lateral pterygoid muscle, c: inferior lateral pterygoid muscle, d: posterior ligaments and retrodiscal tissues, e: condyle, f: inferior joint space, g: superior joint space, h: perforation through posterior ligament, i. **B.** Dye in inferior joint space only. **C.** Leakage of dye through a perforation(*arrow*) in the posterior ligament. Notice how dye then spreads into superior joint space

9.3.6 Treating Complete Disk Displacement

9. 3. 6. 1 Treatment categories

For treatment purposes, the various conditions of complete disk displacement can be categorized into treatment groups:

(1) Complete anterior disk displacement

1) Reducible to function.

2) Segmentally reducible to function.

3) Reducible but not maintainable in function.

4) Nonreducible, repairable.

5) Nonreducible, nonrepairable.

(2) Posterior disk displacement

By extending the diagnosis to further define the various conditions that exist within the broad group of anteriorly displaced disks. You can target treatment toward specific conditions rather than using a broad-spectrum nonspecific treatment for all displaced disks. The need for this type of specificity becomes apparent in a practice that sees a large number of patients with TMDs. It is not uncommon to see patients wearing anterior repositioning splints for the purpose of capturing ankylosed, nonrepairable, or even nonexistent disks. Such erroneous, empiric treatment has no chance for success. If the exact purpose of the prescribed treatment is not targeted at a clearly defined condition, the diagnosis is incomplete.

9. 3. 6. 2 Complete anterior disk displacement, reducible to function

Treatment for displaced disks that are reducible to function should have three objectives that must be fulfilled:

① Recapture of the disk in correct alignment

② Translation of the condyle to centric relation without loss of the recaptured disk

③ Maintenance of correct disk alignment in function

9. 3. 6. 3 Complete anterior disc displacement, reducible but not maintainable in function

Being able to recapture a displaced disk does not necessarily mean it will stay recaptured during function. There are three types of disk problems that may prevent maintaining alignment through the functional range of condylar movement:

(1) Hypermobility of the disk.

(2) Hypomobility of the disk.

(3) Deformity of the disk.

9. 3. 6. 4 Complete anterior disk displacement, nonreducible but repairable

The options for nonreducible disk displacements are narrowed down to two:

(1) Surgical correction or repair.

(2) Using the patient's adaptive response.

Anterior repositioning devices have no vale for a noncapturable disk. In fact, they are contraindicated. The purpose of anterior repositioning is to unload the retrodiscal tissues so that they can heal and regain the elastic traction necessary for pulling the disk back with the condyle. We pay a price for anterior repositioning because it produces muscle incoordination. Whenever the mandible is displaced forward of centric relation (even when it is intentional), the combination of lateral pterygoid bracing against elevator muscle contraction occurs. Incoordinated antagonistic muscle contraction has a tendency to develop into muscle hypercontraction. So unless that hypercontraction is directed through the disk, the loading is applied onto the very tissues we are trying to heal. If beneficial adaptive changes are to be encouraged in the retrodiscal tissues, they will occur more readily with the decreased in muscle loading of a peaceful neuromuscular harmony. We do not achieve a peaceful neuromusculature with anterior repositioning forward of medial pole bracing by bone.

If the disk is nonreducible, the first treatment decision whether recapture of the disk is essential for an acceptable

The use of an anterior bite plane is a practical and effective muscle-relaxation splint to use in combination with TMJ surgery for correction of a displaced disk. Eliminating all posterior occlusal stops may seem like an odd way to reduce the load on the joint, but it works very effectively because of the effect of posterior disclusion on elevator muscle contraction. Posterior disclusion causes two of the three elevator muscles to release and thus reduces muscular loading of the joint. The procedure has the added advantage of being easier to fabricate before surgery. Postoperative adjustment is simplified because only the anterior teeth contact. As soon as reasonable joint stability is confirmed, the appliance should be converted to a full occlusal splint to prevent supraeruption of the posterior teeth. Periodic adjustment of the splint should continue until minimal or no ad-

justment is needed. AL that point, final occlusal treatment can be completed if needed.

9. 3. 6. 5 Complete anterior disk displacement, nonreducible and nonrepairable

The disk may become irreparably displaced because of damage to either the disk itself or the ligaments that attach it to the condyle and the temporal bone.

Destruction of the disk can occur when it is folded, bunched up, or torn so that subsequent loading leads to disintegration or noncorrectable misshaping.

Microsurgical reparative techniques continue to improve. Today there are very few damaged disks that cannot be reshaped and repaired, but there are some that are unquestionably unsalvageable. Most nonrepairable disks are found in older patients, and in many cases the adaptive process will have already changed the contours of the articular surfaces before you see the patient for examination.

9. 3. 6. 6 Inflammatory degenerative joint disease (osteoarthritis)

Inflammation appears to be a secondary sequela to unstabilized remodeling of bony surfaces that are overloaded.

Gross changes in the articular surfaces can be expected to match the meniscus displacement and its altered shape. If the primary soft tissues change shape, the secondary (bone) tissues adapt. If the primary tissues can be corrected in time, corrective reshaping of secondary tissues can occur as a normal process of adaptive remodeling. If the displaced soft tissues cannot be repaired, the remodeling process continues to adapt the shape of the articular surfaces to conform to the surfaces they load against. The process progresses continuously after the onset of disk displacement. Whether the remodeling process remains a reparative adaptive response or becomes a degenerative disease depends on the combined factors of host resistance and the degree of bruxing or clenching that determines the intensity of load that the bony surfaces must resist. Severe bruxing or clenching when the disk is displaced will most certainly lead to flattening of the condyle and often the eminentia. If the load is greater than the adaptive capacity for conformative remodeling, inflammatory degenerative changes start to occur. Degenerative joint disease varies from patient to patient and is affected by general factors of health, nutrition, and body chemistry changes such as those occurring with hormonal imbalances.

Even in severely flattened condyle and eminentia contours, however, it is possible to have a reasonable degree of stability and an acceptable level of comfort. This depends on the character of the remodeled bone surfaces, which in some instances form very hard smooth surfaces referred to as eburnated bone.

Radiographically, the trabeculas in eburnated bone are densely packed and the articular surfaces have the appearance of cortical bone. The severe flattening of the articular surfaces is evidence that the disk is absent. The bone-to-bone contact of the condyle against the eminentia is evidence on properly angulated transcranial films. Radiographs should be taken in both the superior hinge position and the opened (protrusive) position to observe the comparative condyle position in function.

Doppler auscultation of the TMI for bone-to-bone contact generates a chirping crepitus that often sounds like a gate swinging on rusty hinges. The crepitation can be rather coarse depending on the roughness of the surfaces that rub. If the fibrocartilage that covers the articular surfaces is still present, the Doppler sounds are less coarse, an indication of articular surfaces that are smoother. As those surfaces break down, the sounds generated are more gravelly.

Axiographic recordings present a protrusive path that is often much flatter and less angulated than the typical convex path. This is an important observation because an abnormally flat condylar path may not be able to disclude the posterior teeth in protrusive excursion. Alteration of the anterior guidance may be necessary to prevent posterior occlusal interferences in the functional ranges.

9. 3. 6. 7   Clinical observations

The complete displacement of the disk almost invariably leads to progressive flattening of the condyle unless the retrodiscal tissues adapt to form a new pad of fibrous tissue. Flattening occurs as a result of loading the condyle against the eminentia without the biconcave disk interposed to maintain the rounded shape of the condyle. If both the condyle and the eminentia are flattened, it is a sign that the overload on the joint occurs through its range of function. Such a functional overload is particularly damaging to the articular surfaces because without the disk present, the lubrication and nutrition from synovial fluids are also lost. Thus the surfaces of the

articulating bones gradually break down, causing a loss of height of the condyle. This loss of height appears to be progressive whenever the disk is lost, And it leads to a further progressive problem of maintaining occlusal harmony.

Because all elevator muscles are behind the teeth, any loss of condylar height causes the upward migration of the condyle to load the most posterior tooth. The damaging effect of such a posterior occlusal pivot is compounded because it separates the anterior teeth and prevents them from fulfilling their job of discluding the posterior teeth in eccentric movements. The result is muscle hypercontraction that overloads both the TMJs and the occlusion. So the joint that is already compromised by loss of its disk is also subjected to the increased loading from the musculature. The problem is progressive because the more the condyle flattens, the more the load is applied to the occlusion.

Perhaps the most dramatic clinical evidence that TMJ problems cannot be separated from occlusal problems can be verified by a consistent observation: Severe wear of upper molar lingual cusps is virtually never seen without also finding commensurate changes in the shape of the condyles or the eminentiae, or both. Nor is severe flattening of the condyle and eminentia observed without directly related occlusal wear. Mongini has shown that changes in condylar shape are directly related to wear patterns in the occlusion and vice versa. If one remembers that maximum muscle contraction does not occur until the teeth are together, it will be obvious that loading of the condyles occurs at that jaw position that relates to maximum intercuspal contact.

9. 3. 6. 8   Treatment

Because loss of the disk also reduces the nutrition and lubrication to the joint surfaces, it does not seem possible to completely stop all degenerative breakdown on the articular surfaces when the disk is missing. Nevertheless, an acceptable comfort level can usually be achieved with a manageable degree of stability if muscle incoordination can be corrected. The adaptive process can favorably alter even a bone-to-bone relationship in most patients if the nearly continuous loading on the joint can be reduced to intermittent loading with reduced intensity. That is the goal of treatment, and it can usually be achieved by correction of the occlusion to make it noninterfering to the superior hinge position of the condyles.

When the disk is missing, the superior hinge

position is determined by bone-to-bone bracing at the medial pole simultaneous with contact against the eminentia. Even in severely flattened condyles, the medial pole of the condyle is still capable of stopping the upward translation of the condyle against the eminentiae. At the bone-braced superior position, the lateral pterygoid muscles can release contraction and allow the elevator muscles to seat the condyles without antagonistic muscle bracing. Even though the disk is missing, muscle coordination can still be achieved if the condyle is free to slide to the superior position without interference from the teeth. The position should be tested for comfort while loading occurs with bilateral pressure. If multiple centric relation stops of equal intensity can be achieved along with immediate disclusion of all posterior contacts in eccentric movement, muscle coordination can be established. Of course, centric relation must be defined differently if there is no disk present. It becomes simply "the most superior position" of the condyles against the eminentiae. This position is labeled adapted centric posture.

Harmonization of the occlusion may be accomplished provisionally on a full occlusal bite splint, or it may be accomplished directly through equilibration. It is a common misconception that when dentitions have been worn flat, there are no occlusal interferences. If both condyles are positioned on their most superior axis against the eminentiae, there will invariably be premature contacts as well as posterior interferences in eccentric pathways (in untreated patients).

If the condylar path has become too flat to work out lateral or protrusive disclusion of the posterior teeth by equilibration, it may be necessary to restore the anterior teeth to provide a disclusive anterior guidance angle. Equilibration should be completed first to eliminate all centric-relation interferences, and then eccentric excursions should be adjusted as far as possible before the anterior guidance is altered. The steeper anterior guidance will interfere with the extremely flattened envelope of function that the patient has developed, so there will be a tendency to brux against the steeper inclines. This does not create any problems of discomfort as a rule, but it does subject the anterior teeth to lateral forces that could be damaging. The best rule is to steepen the anterior guidance only as much as necessary to adequately disclude the posterior teeth in all excursions, allowing for some eventual wear of the anteri-

or inclines.

The most important occlusal change to make when the disk is irreparably displaced is to provide disclusion of all posterior teeth in all mandibular positions except centric relation. This always involves the anterior guidance as a disclusive factor. The main purpose of this occlusal relationship is the reduction of elevator muscle loading on the condyles. This reduction occurs when posterior teeth disclude. I have found that providing this type of occlusal function noticeably reduces the amount and frequency of postoperative occlusal corrections needed for patients with no disks.

Patients should be made aware that periodic correction of the occlusion will be necessary to keep the neuromuscular system as peaceful as possible. When the disk has been lost, some degenerative changes seem to occur continuously on the articular surfaces regardless of treatment. Maintaining occlusal harmony reduces the changes to a manageable level. An occlusal splint, processed in acrylic resin, is often helpful in reducing the amount of wear on the teeth. It should be adjusted for simultaneous, equal intensity stops on all teeth in adapted centric posture and for disclusion of posterior teeth in all eccentric positions. Most patients are able to maintain the occlusal surfaces reasonably free of extensive wear just by wearing the appliance at night.

9.3.6.9   Inflammatory degenerative joint disease (osteoarthritis)

When the load applied through the condyle is greater than the patient's adaptive capacity for remodeling to occur without inflammation, the articular cartilage breaks down, and soft, vascular tissue invades the articular surfaces. All bearing surfaces may be involved, including the disk if it is still present. The joint may become painful as the loss of the articular cartilage exposes sensory nerves. Condylar height may be lost, sometimes rather suddenly, thereby intensifying occlusal disharmony and its resultant muscle incoordination. I have not seen a single patient with active osteoarthritis of the TMJ who did not present with concomitant masticatory muscle tenderness when palpated.

Bilateral loading of the joints produces a range of discomfort from tenderness to sharp pain. It is usually this response to routine testing of the joints that first alerts us to the possibility of intra-articular pathosis, which then must be confirmed by radiographic methods.

Lesions in the articular surfaces can usually be seen on transcranial films, but a panoramic radiograph sometimes gives a better image. If a lesion cannot be confirmed by either method in a suspected osteoarthritis joint, a submental vertex view may be used to locate it in some instances. The most reliable method, however, for a laminar assessment of the joint surfaces is CT. A TMJ that cannot resist loading without discomfort should be analyzed with progressively more specific methods until the source of discomfort is determined. CT and nuclear magnetic resonance imaging both have value in the search for a verified diagnosis in certain cases and may be selected on the basis of specific need.

The onset of osteoarthritis in the TMJ is apparently more complex than can be explained solely by muscular overload. There appears to be a greater tendency for the disease in females, but at least clinically there also appears to be an increased predisposition for symptoms related to muscle incoordination in women. The role that hormonal imbalance plays could be directed toward disturbances in calcium metabolism that affect both bone and muscle function, so that too could be a factor. The common finding of osteoarthritis occurring unilaterally raises some doubts about a generalized metabolic factor as the principal cause and seems to indicate that host resistance is more of a contributing factor. Despite the role that various contributing factors appear to play in the onset of the inflammatory stage, osteoarthritis does not appear to be initiated in the absence of an overload. Furthermore, the reduction of the load on the damaged joint seems to stop the pathosis and stimulate regenerative remodeling. If the disk is intact enough to be repaired or repositioned, the remodeling occurs more rapidly and may even recontour the condyle back to a normal convex shape. The remodeled joint contour depends on the contour of the surface that it functions against; so if the disk is absent, the condyle may adapt itself to a flattened surface, but functional harmony can still be achieved in most instances if muscular overload can be reduced sufficiently.

When active osteoarthritis is observed, the finalization of occlusal surfaces should not be attempted. Until the pathosis is stopped and the defect repaired, the superior axis position cannot be determined with certainty. It then becomes necessary to work with a tentative treatment position. Full occlusal splint offer the best choice for the progressive adjustment of the occlusion as the condyle's position

changes during its adaptive remodeling. After the joint stabilizes to a point that requires only minimal occlusal adjustment, occlusal surfaces can be restored. If the disk is absent, the best result that can be achieved will not completely stop all the generation at the articular surfaces, but it can usually be slowed to a level that allows occluso-muscle adjustment. Nighttime use of a full occlusal splint can help in this maintenance effort.

The above depiction of intracapsular TMDs is a very "usefriendly" analysis of what practicing clinicians find in everyday practice. Understanding how the variability of disk misalignment affects clinical decisions regarding occlusal diagnosis and treatment is extremely important, and the explanations given will serve clinicians well. It is also recommended that the guidelines prepared by The American society of Temporomandibular Joint Surgeons should be studied on their website for a more complete coverage of specific types and subtypes of TMDs.

9.4　Classification of Intracapsular Disorders

9.4.1　*Principle*
Treatment selection depends on the specific classification of the disorder to be treated.

9.4.2　*Practical Temporomandibular Joint Analysis*
To have practical value in clinical practice, a classification system for the condition of the temporomandibular joints (TMJs) must be based on objective findings. It must be simple enough to use that it can be a standard, cost-effective, and time-effective part of every complete examination. In spite of its simplicity, Piper's classification is complete in all the necessary details for TMJ examination. It is specific in its precise analysis of the intracapsular structures, making it the recommended "gold standard" for research as well as for everyday clinical practice.

Before any treatment is selected, it is important to classify the specific type of temporomandibular disorder (TMD) into:
　(1) Occluso-muscle disorder.
　(2) Intracapsular disorders.
　(3) Disorders that mimic TMDs.

9.4.3　*Systemized Approach to Classification*
The system we have adopted for intracapsular dis-

order is the classification by Piper. This classification has become the gold standard, and it is the most practical system for clarifying the exact condition of the TMJs. It describes TMDs in relation to the progressive patterns of deformation in specific intracapsular structures that have a profound effect on occlusion as well as symptoms of orofacial and TMJ pain.

The stages, as described, form a matrix of signs and symptoms that can be determined with specificity by using a series of testing procedures. A diagnosis must be considered inadequate if it merely states that there is a reciprocal click, or if it states that a displaced disk is reducible or nonreducible without differentiation of whether the disk is completely displaced or partially displaced off the lateral pole only.

In evaluating any TMD, disk alignment on the medial pole and the lateral pole must be evaluated separately.

If the medial pole can maintain an acceptable alignment with the disk, the long-term prognosis is quite good for successfully establishing a harmonious occlusion and a peaceful neuromusculature with complete relief of pain. This favorable prognosis is achievable in most patients even if the lateral pole disk relationship is a closed lock that is not reducible.

Diagnosis of TMDs is not based on observation of a single factor. Proper diagnosis requires a combination of tests that must be related to key questions in the history. The value of Piper's classification system is that it uses objective tests for evaluating specific structures, so there is no need to rely solely on patients' subjective descriptions of their symptoms. The key to effective diagnosis then becomes a testing process to determine the structural basis for each sign or symptom.

Anatomic and histologic classifications of TMDs provide the most useful mechanism for tracking stages of disease and potential treatment options.

The classification of TMJ condition directs what you should do for each patient. It guides you in the information you give your patient, and it warns you in advance against starting treatment that could be problematic. Classification of a TMJ condition is an essential part of every new patient examination.

■ Summary

The summary of the chapter is the pathogenesis of TMD, and the relationship between the occlusion, muscle, intracapsular disorders and TMD. The pathogenesis, description, methods of diagnosis and treatment of each disorders will be introduced.

■ Questions

1. What is the main pathogenesis of the temporomandibular disorders?
2. What are the main treatment methods of the temporomandibular disorders?

(Xiaojiang Yang   杨晓江)

References

[1] Belser U, Hannam AC. The influence of altered working-side occlusal guidance on masticatory muscles and related jaw movement. J Prosthet Dent,1985,53(3):406-413.
[2] Dawson PE. Centric relation: Its effect on occluso-muscle harmony. Dent Clin North Am, 1979,23(2):169-180.
[3] Dawson PE. Position paper: regarding diagnosis, management, and treatment of temporomandibular disorders. J Prosthet Dent, 1999,81(2):174-178.
[4] Dawson PE. Temporomandibular joint pain-dysfunction problems can be solved. J Prosthet Dent, 1973,29(1):100-112.
[5] Hannam AC, De Cou RE, Scott JD, et al. The relationship between dental occlusion, muscle activity, and associated jaw movements in man. Arch Oral Biol Arch Oral Biol,1977,22(1):25-32.
[6] Ingervall B, Carlsson GE. Masticatory muscle activity before and after elimination of balancing side occlusal interferences. J Oral Rehab,1982,9(3):183-192.
[7] Kerstein RB,Farrell S. Treatment of myofascial pain-dysfunction syndrome with occlusal equilibration. J Prosthet Dent,1990,63(6):695-700.
[8] Kerstein RB. Treatment of myofascial pain dysfunction syndrome with occlusal therapy to reduce lengthy disclusion time-a recall study. Cranio, 1995,13(2):105-115.
[9] Kerveskari P, Bell L, Salonen M, et al. Effect of elimination of occlusal interferences on sighs and symptoms of craniomandibular disorders in young adult. J Oral Rehabil, 1989,16(1):21-26.
[10] Krough Poulson WG, Olsson A. Occlusal disharmonies and dysfunction of the stomatognathic system. Dent Clin NA,1966,11:627-635.
[11] Mahan P. Pathologic manifestations of occlusal disharmo-

ny. New York: Continuum, 1981:87-98.

[12] Riise C, Sheikholeslam A. The influence of experimental interfering occlusal contacts on postural activity of the anterior temporal and masseter muscles in young adults. J Oral Rehabil,1982,9(5):419-425.

[13] Schaerer P, Stallard RE, Zander HA. Occlusal interferences and mastication: an electromyographic study. J Prosthet Dent,1967,17(5):438-449.

[14] Tarantola GJ, Becker IM, Gremillion H, et al. The effectiveness of equilibration in the improvement of signs and symptoms in the stomatognathic system. Int J Perio Rest Dent,1998,18(6):594-603.

[15] Chuong R, Piper MA. Open reduction of condylar fractures of the mandible in conjunction with repair of discal injury: A preliminary report. J Oral Maxillofac Surg, 1988,46(4):257-263.

Chapter

10

Maxillofacial Pathology

▪ Objectives

The objective of the chapter is to provide an overview of maxillofacial pathology including odontogenic diseases, salivary diseases, premalignant diseases and oral cancer. Its target audiences are undergraduate and postgraduate students as well as practitioners.

▪ Key concepts

The maxillofacial region is composed of jaw bones, oral mucosa, teeth and a variety of salivary glands. So the diseases in maxillofacial region can be classified depending on the tissues from which the diseases originated. Odontogenic diseases are common lesions in the jaw bone. Oral cancer and premalignant lesions originated from oral mucosa. The salivary diseases includes a variety of adenomas.

▪ Introduction

One of the major roles of the oral and maxillofacial surgeon is that of diagnostician. From private practices in small communities to large tertiary care medical centers, these specialists are called upon to evaluate and diagnose a wide variety of conditions affecting the face, jaws, head, and neck as well as the tissues of the oral cavity. An accurate diagnosis is obviously important and occasionally critical to the patient so that the most appropriate treatment can be initiated as soon as possible. Early determination of the true diagnosis can further benefit the patient by avoiding the need for expensive unnecessary laboratory studies, the use of ineffective or improper medications, and the inconvenience of additional costly consultation(s).

Odontogenic Diseases

10. 1. 1   *Odontogenic Cysts*

With rare exceptions, epithelium-lined cysts in bone are seen only in the jaws. Other than a few cysts that may result from the inclusion of epithelium along embryonic lines of fusion, most jaw cysts are lined by epithelium that is derived from odontogenic epithelium, hence the term **odontogenic cysts.** These cysts are subclassified as developmental or inflammatory in nature. Although the cell type is often known, developmental cysts are of unknown origin; however, they do not seem to be the result of an inflammatory reaction. Inflammatory cysts, on the other hand, are the result of inflammation.

10. 1. 1. 1   Dentigerous cyst

By definition, a dentigerous cyst occurs in association with an unerupted tooth, most commonly mandibular third molars. Other common associations are with maxillary third molars, maxillary canines, and mandibular second premolars. They may also occur around supernumerary teeth and in association with odontomas; however, they are only rarely associated with primary teeth. Although dentigerous cysts occur over a wide age range, they are most commonly seen in 10- to 30-year old. Many dentigerous cysts are small asymptomatic lesions that are discovered serendipitously on routine radiographs, although some may grow to considerable size causing bony expansion that is usually painless until secondary infection occurs.

Radiographically, the dentigerous cyst presents as a well-defined unilocular radiolucency, often with a sclerotic border. Since the epithelial lining is derived from the reduced enamel epithelium, this radiolucency typically and preferentially surrounds the crown of the tooth. A large dentigerous cyst may give the impression of a multilocular process because of the persistence of bone trabeculae within the radiolucency. However, dentigerous cysts are grossly and histopathologically unilocular processes and probably are never truly multilocular lesions. Three types of dentigerous cyst have been described radiographically, including the **central** variety, in which the radiolucency surrounds just the crown of the tooth, with the crown projecting into the cyst lumen. In the **lateral** variety, the cyst develops laterally along the tooth root and partially surrounds the crown. The

circumferential variant of the dentigerous cyst exists when the cyst surrounds the crown but also extends down along the root surface, as if the entire tooth were located within the cyst.

One diagnostic dilemma is distinguishing between a dentigerous cyst and an enlarged dental follicle. This distinction becomes clinically significant when the surgeon considers whether to submit tissue removed with an impacted third molar for histopathologic examination as opposed to clinical designation as a follicle, with simple disposal of the tissue. The radiographic distinction becomes somewhat arbitrary; however, any pericoronal radiolucency that is > 4 or 5 mm is considered suggestive of cyst formation and should be submitted for microscopic examination. It is noteworthy that pathologists also struggle with the distinction between dental follicles associated with developing teeth and odontogenic lesions. It seems that odontogenic cysts, odontogenic fibroma, and odontogenic myxoma are the lesions most often inappropriately diagnosed by surgical pathologists owing to a general unfamiliarity with the normal process of odontogenesis.

Of perhaps even greater concern is the large unilocular radiolucency. Although most commonly classified radiographically as dentigerous cysts, it is incumbent upon the surgeon to section these excised specimens in the operating room and to consider frozen-section analysis. In fact, some specimens may contain a focus of unicystic ameloblastoma and therefore require consideration of more extensive treatment.

The histologic features of dentigerous cysts may vary greatly depending mainly on whether or not the cyst is inflamed. In the noninflamed dentigerous cyst, a thin epithelial lining may be present with the fibrous connective tissue wall loosely arranged. In the inflamed dentigerous cyst, the epithelium commonly demonstrates hyperplastic rete ridges, and the fibrous cyst wall shows an inflammatory infiltrate.

Most dentigerous cysts are treated with enucleation of the cyst and removal of the associated tooth, often without a preceding incisional biopsy. Larger cysts that are treated in the operating room should probably undergo frozen-section diagnosis and appropriate treatment that might be dictated by other diagnoses. Curettage of the cyst cavity is usually advisable at the time of removal of the cyst in the event that a more aggressive cyst is diagnosed histopathologically following removal in an office setting. Such diagnoses would include odontogenic keratocyst and unicystic ameloblastoma.

Large dentigerous cysts may be treated with marsupialization when enucleation and curettage might otherwise result in neurosensory dysfunction or predispose the patient to an increased chance of pathologic fracture. Some patients who are not candidates for general anesthesia may also be treated with a marsupialization procedure in an office setting under local anesthesia. This permits decompression of the large dentigerous cyst with a resultant reduction in the size of the cyst and bony defect. At a later date the reduced cyst can be removed in a smaller-scale surgery.

The need is emphasized for histopathologic examination of all radiolucencies that are empirically diagnosed as dentigerous cysts. This includes those that are enucleated as well as those that undergo marsupialization, during which it is important to inspect the cyst lumen and submit a representative piece for histopathologic examination. Support of this statement stems from the occasional formation of a squamous cell carcinoma, mucoepidermoid carcinoma, or ameloblastoma from or in association with a dentigerous cyst. The prognosis for most histopathologically diagnosed dentigerous cysts is excellent, with recurrence being a rare finding.

10. 1. 1. 2 Odontogenic keratocyst

The odontogenic keratocyst is a distinctive form of developmental odontogenic cyst that deserves special consideration because of its specific histopathologic features and aggressive clinical behavior. Two variants of this cyst are well known; the sporadic cyst and the cyst associated with the nevoid basal cell carcinoma syndrome. Both variants of the odontogenic keratocyst are believed to be derived from remnants of the dental lamina. This cyst shows a different growth mechanism and biologic behavior from the previously described dentigerous cyst. Most authors believe that dentigerous cysts continue to enlarge as a result of increased osmotic pressure within the lumen of the cyst. This mechanism does not appear to hold true for odontogenic keratocysts, and their growth may be related to unknown factors inherent in the epithelium itself of enzymatic activity in the fibrous wall.

Adequate diagnosis and treatment of the odontogenic keratocyst is important for three reasons: ① this cyst is recognized as being more aggressive than other odontogenic cysts, ② the odontogenic keratocyst has a higher rate of recurrence than other odontogenic cysts, and ③ the association with nevoid basal cell carcinoma syndrome requires that the clinician examine a patient with multiple cysts of the jaws for physical findings that might diagnose this syndrome.

Odontogenic keratocysts may be found in patients ranging in age from infancy to old age; however, 60% of cases are seen in people between 10 and 40 years old. A slight male predilection is usually seen, and 60% to 80% of cases involve the mandible, particularly in the posterior body and ascending ramus. Although it is rare for a dentigerous cyst to appear multilocular on radiographs, it is most common for odontogenic keratocysts to appear multilocular. Many appear unilocular and can therefore be confused with dentigerous cysts. It is clear, therefore, that the differential diagnosis of a unilocular radiolucency must include both entities and that treatment should include curettage in the event that the diagnosis is odontogenic keratocyst. When multiple multilocular radiolucencies are noted on a panoramic radiograph, the clinician must perform an incisional biopsy and investigate the possibility of nevoid basal cell carcinoma syndrome.

Histologically, the odontogenic keratocyst is readily recognized. A uniform layer of stratified squamous epithelium, usually six to eight cells in thickness, is present. The parakeratotic surface is characteristically corrugated. The wall is usually thin and friable, which can pose problems for removal in one piece intraoperatively. Epithelial budding and the presence of daughter cysts may be noted in the connective tissue wall. It is generally advisable to ask the pathologist to examine the sections carefully for these two features as they generally impart a more aggressive character to the cyst.

Like the treatment of most odontogenic cysts, the odontogenic keratocyst may be treated with enucleation and curettage and must be removed in one piece, which requires acceptable access and lighting. As such, many patients are suitably treated in an operating room setting under general anesthesia. This is particularly helpful when removing large cysts. It is my experience and that of others that a large majority of sporadic odontogenic keratocysts may be effectively managed with a thorough enucleation and curettage surgery. Macintosh has advocated the resection of odontogenic keratocysts with 5 mm linear margins as the preferred primary method of treatment, and has reported on 37 patients with 43 lesions emphasizing the efficacy and superior results of resection over all other therapeutic undertakings.

The reported frequency of recurrence of the odontogenic keratocyst ranges from 2.5% to 62.5% in various studies. This wide variation may be related to the total number of cases studied, the length of follow-up periods, and the inclusion or exclusion of orthokeratinized cysts in the study group. Several reports that include large numbers of cases indicate a recurrence rate of approximately 30%. Regezi and colleagues point out that the recurrence rate for solitary odontogenic keratocysts is 10% to 30%. They indicate that approximately 5% of patients with odontogenic keratocysts have multiple sporadic jaw cysts (nonsyndromic) and that their recurrence rate is greater than that for solitary lesions. Brannon has suggested three mechanisms responsible for recurrence: ① remnants of dental lamina within the jaws not associated with the original odontogenic keratocyst being responsible for de novo cyst formation; ② incomplete removal (persistence) of the original cyst secondary to a thin friable lining and cortical perforation with adherence to adjacent soft tissue; and ③ remaining rests of dental lamina and satellite cysts following enucleation. Vedtofte and Praetorius reviewed 72 patients with 75 odontogenic keratocysts and observed remnants of dental lamina between the cyst membrane and overlying mucosa. As such, they advocated the excision of overlying mucosa in conjunction with removal of the cyst. Williams and Connor recommended a primary enucleation and curettage surgery for odontogenic keratocysts, including the use of methylene blue as a marking agent, followed by a 3-minute application of Carnoy's solution. They indicated that resection should be considered for the treatment of a recurrent odontogenic keratocyst, with inclusion of appropriate bone and soft tissue margins.

Pathogenetically, the odontogenic keratocyst expresses cell cycle phenomena that support its proliferation. These include the release of the cytokines interleukin 1a (IL-1a) and IL-6 as well as parathyroid hormone-related protein that encourage resorption of bone. Moreover, the expression of proliferating cell nuclear antigen (PCNA) in odontogenic cysts has been assessed. It is hypothesized that the identification of the proliferative activity in odontogenic cysts and tumors may be useful to predict their biologic behavior. The same may be true of the Ki-67 antigen. In fact, two studies have been performed that have quantified these parameters. The conclusion of both studies is that an increased proliferative activity for the odontogenic keratocyst in comparison with the dentigerous cyst is noted consistently. These results are in agreement with the more aggressive behavior seen with the odontogenic keratocyst.

The orthokeratinized odontogenic cyst, once thought to be a variant of the odontogenic keratocyst, is now generally well accepted as being a different clinicopathologic entity from the more common parakeratinized odontogenic keratocyst; it should therefore be placed in a different category. These cysts usually appear as unilocular radiolucencies, but occasional examples have been multilocular. A majority of these cysts are encountered in a lesion that appears clinically and radiographically to represent a dentigerous cyst, most often involving an unerupted mandibular third molar tooth. Histologically, the epithelium is thin and orthokeratinized, and a prominent palisaded basal layer, characteristic of the odontogenic keratocyst, is not present. Enucleation and curettage of the orthokeratinized cyst is curative in most cases. The reported rate of recurrence of 2% is far lower than the previously quoted statistics for recurrence of the odontogenic keratocyst.

10.1.1.3 Nevoid basal cell carcinoma syndrome

The nevoid basal cell carcinoma syndrome (basal cell nevus syndrome, Gorlin's syndrome) is an autosomal-dominant inherited condition that exhibits high penetrance and variable expressivity. It is caused by mutations in the *PTCH* tumor suppressor gene, mapped to chromosome 9q22.3-q31. Affected patients may demonstrate frontal and temporoparietal bossing, hypertelorism, and mandibular prognathism. Other frequent skeletal anomalies include bifid ribs and lamellar calcification of the falx cerebri. The most significant clinical feature is the tendency to develop multiple basal cell carcinomas that may affect both exposed and non-sun-exposed areas of the skin. Pitting defects on the palms and soles can be found in nearly two-thirds of affected patients. The discovery of multiple odontogenic keratocysts is usually the first manifestation of the syndrome that leads to the diagnosis. For this reason, any patient with an odontogenic keratocyst should be evaluated for this condition. Although the cysts in patients with nevoid basal cell carcinoma syndrome cannot definitely be distinguished microscopically from those not associated with the syndrome, they often demonstrate more epithelial proliferation and daughter cyst formation in the cyst wall.

The treatment of the odontogenic keratocyst in patients with nevoid basal cell carcinoma syndrome can be difficult owing to the large number of "recurrences" in these patients. As a matter of point, I choose to refer to these as new primary cysts owing to the autosomaldominant penetrance of the syndrome and cyst development. It is certainly possible that many of these cysts are persistent, particularly when considering how common it can be to retain rests of the dental lamina when enucleating an odontogenic keratocyst. Whatever the mechanism, a resection hardly seems to be warranted. Marsupialization is a more desirable procedure and has been shown to result in complete resolution of the sporadic cyst, with no histologic signs of cystic remnants, daughter cysts, or budding of the basal layer of the epithelium. Although all of the eight cases in the series by Pogrel and Jordan were sporadic cysts, a similar approach to syndrome patients with odontogenic keratocysts that had been operated on multiple times has been performed with success in a small sample size.

10.1.2 Odontogenic Tumors

The ameloblastoma is the most common clinically significant and potentially lethal odontogenic tumor. Excluding odontomas, its incidence equals or exceeds the combined total of all other odontogenic tumors. These tumors may arise from rests of the dental lamina, a developing enamel organ, the epithelial lining of an odontogenic cyst, or the basal cells of the oral mucosa. The ameloblastoma occurs in three different variants, each with specific implications for treatment and a unique prognosis: solid or multicystic, unicystic, and peripheral. In an analysis of the international literature, 3,677 cases of ameloblastoma were reviewed, of which 92% were solid or multicystic, 6% were unicystic, and 2% were peripheral.

10.1.2.1   Solid or multicystic ameloblastoma

This variant of the ameloblastoma is encountered in patients over a wide age range. It is rare in children in their first decade of life and relatively uncommon in the second decade. The tumor shows a relatively equal rate of occurrence in the third through seventh decades. There is no gender predilection, and racial predilection is most controversial. About 85% of this variant of the ameloblastoma occur in the mandible, most commonly in the molar/ramus region. About 15% of multicystic ameloblastomas occur in the maxilla, usually in the posterior regions. A painless expansion of the jaws is the most common clinical presentation; neurosensory changes are uncommon, even with large tumors. Slow growth is the rule, with untreated tumors leading to tremendous facial disfigurement.

The most common radiographic feature is that of a multilocular radiolucency. Buccal and lingual cortical expansion is common, frequently to the point of perforation. Resorption of adjacent tooth roots is common. Histologic patterns include **follicular**, in which the stellate reticulum is located within the center of the odontogenic island; **plexiform**, in which the stellate reticulum is located outside of the odontogenic rest; **acanthomatous**, in which squamous differentiation of the odontogenic epithelium is present; **granular cell**, in which the tumor islands exhibit cells that demonstrate abundant granular eosinophilic cytoplasm; **desmoplastic** owing to extremely dense collagenized stroma that supports the tumor; and the least common **basal cell** variant, in which nests of uniform basaloid cells are present, with a strong resemblance to basal cell carcinoma. In this latter tumor stellate reticulum is not present in the central portions of the nests. One additional exception surrounds the desmoplastic variant, which is generally not a radiolucent tumor radiographically owing to its high content of collagenized stroma.

Pathogenetically, the proliferative capacity of ameloblastomas has been studied. As might be conjectured, the recurrent ameloblastoma is associated with the highest number of PCNA-positive cells, followed by the previously unoperated ameloblastomas. The nuclear PCNA positivity of the unicystic ameloblastoma was notably lower than the positivity of the solid multicystic ameloblastoma. Other cell cycle features supporting the aggressive behavior of the ameloblastoma include the overexpression of *BCL*2 and *BCLX*, as well as the expression of IL-1 and IL-6.

The ameloblastoma continues to be a subject of fascination in the international literature. Unfortunately, although most agree that aggressive treatment is essential for cure of this tumor, the fact remains that a consensus has not been reached on the biologic behavior of this neoplasm and how best to treat it. The literature is therefore paradoxically a source of both information and misinformation. Conflicting opinion, extending backward in time, has served both to educate and to confuse, and it has been left to generations of surgeons to sift and interpret what they consider to be clinically valid. It is my strong opinion that this neoplasm is both highly aggressive and curable. This notwithstanding, numerous methods of treatment have been recommended, ranging from simple enucleation and curettage to resection.

The solid or multicystic ameloblastoma tends to infiltrate between intact cancellous bone trabeculae at the periphery of the tumor before bone resorption becomes radiographically evident. Therefore, the actual margin of the tumor often extends beyond its apparent radiographic or clinical margin. 60 Attempts to remove the tumor by curettage, therefore, predictably leave behind small islands of tumor within the bone, which are later determined to be recurrent disease. These must be realized as **persistent disease** as the tumor was never controlled from the outset. When a small burden of tumor is left behind, it may be decades before this persistent disease becomes clinically and radiographically evident, and long after a surgeon falsely proclaimed the patient to be cured.

Owing to the highly infiltrative and aggressive nature of the solid or multicystic ameloblastoma, I recommend resection of the tumor with 1. 0 cm linear bony margins. This linear bony margin should be confirmed by intraoperative specimen radiographs. Soft tissue margins are best managed according to the anatomic barrier margin principles whereby one uninvolved surrounding anatomic barrier is sacrificed on the periphery of the specimen. When all soft and hard tissue margins are histologically negative, the patient is likely to be cured of this neoplasm. Unfortunately, any less aggressive treatment modality may be fraught with inevitable persistence discovered at variable times postoperatively. Moreover, although the persistent and occasionally nonresectable ameloblastoma is radiosensitive, once this otherwise benign tumor defies curative surgical therapy, radiation is of questionable use in salvaging these patients.

10. 1. 2. 2 Unicystic ameloblastoma

In 1970 Vickers and Gorlin published their findings regarding the histologic alterations associated with neoplastic transformation of ameloblastomatous epithelium. These histologic changes were ① hyperchromatism of basal cell nuclei of the epithelium lining the cystic cavities; ② palisading and polarization of basal cell nuclei of the epithelium lining the cystic cavities and ③ cytoplasmic vacuolization, particularly of basal cells of cystic linings. They referred to these changes as early histopathologic features of neoplasia. **Unicystic ameloblastoma** refers to a pattern of epithelial proliferation that has been described in dentigerous cysts of the jaws that does not exhibit the histologic criteria for ameloblastoma published by Vickers and Gorlin. This entity deserves separate consideration based on its clinical, radiographic, and pathologic features. Moreover, in many cases it may be treated more conservatively than the solid or multicystic ameloblastoma with the same degree of cure.

Unicystic ameloblastomas are most commonly seen in young patients, with about 50% of these tumors being diagnosed during the second decade of life. The average age of patients with unicystic ameloblastomas has been reported as 22. 1 years, compared with 40. 2 years for the solid or multicystic variant. More than 90% of these tumors are found in the mandible, usually in the molar/ramus region. A unilocular radiolucency, mimicking a dentigerous cyst, is the most common radiographic presentation for the unicystic ameloblastoma. Most, if not all, unicystic ameloblastomas are unilocular radiolucencies. Three histopathologic variants of unicystic ameloblastoma have been described that impact treatment and prognosis. In the **luminal unicystic ameloblastoma**, the tumor is confined to the luminal surface of the cyst. The lesion consists of a fibrous cyst wall with a lining that consists totally or partially of ameloblastic epithelium. The **intraluminal unicystic ameloblastoma** contains one or more nodules of ameloblastoma projecting from the cystic lining into the lumen of the cyst. These nodules may be relatively small or largely fill the cystic lumen, and are noted to show a plexiform pattern that resembles the plexiform pattern seen in conventional ameloblastomas. As such, these tumors are referred to as plexiform unicystic ameloblastomas. In the third variant, known as **mural unicystic ameloblastoma**, the fibrous wall of the cyst is infiltrated by typical follicular or plexiform ameloblastoma. The extent and depth of the ameloblastic infiltration may vary considerably.

Pathogenetically, the unicystic ameloblastoma seems to have a proliferative capacity between that of the odontogenic keratocyst and the solid or multicystic ameloblastoma.

The clinical and radiographic findings in most cases of unicystic ameloblastoma suggest that the lesion is an odontogenic cyst, most commonly a dentigerous cyst. Under the circumstances the surgeon should routinely open a "cystic" lesion and look for luminal proliferation of tumor. When able, histopathologic examination of such a process should occur with frozen sections. This is particularly important when dealing with large cysts. With a histologic diagnosis of unicystic ameloblastoma, the surgeon should request the pathologist to obtain multiple sections through many levels of the specimen to properly subclassify the variant of unicystic ameloblastoma. When the ameloblastic elements are confined to the lumen of the cyst with or without intraluminal tumor extension, the enucleation has probably been curative treatment. When the cyst wall has been violated by the tumor as in a mural variant of unicystic ameloblastoma, the most appropriate surgical management is quite controversial. If this diagnosis is made postoperatively, the surgeon may wish to adopt close indefinite follow-up examinations of the patient. If a preoperative incisional biopsy provides a diagnosis of mural unicystic ameloblastoma, the surgeon might recommend a resection of the tumor owing to the fact that this variant of the unicystic ameloblastoma has a higher rate of persistence than do the luminal or intraluminal unicystic ameloblastomas.

The treatment of a luminal or intraluminal variant of the unicystic ameloblastoma is enucleation and curettage. In a collective sense, the "recurrence" rate of all unicystic ameloblastomas has been reported as 10% to 20% following enucleation and curettage. This is significantly lower than that of enucleation and curettage of the solid or multicystic ameloblastoma. The question then arises as to when to resect a unicystic ameloblastoma. Three instances are likely to require such treatment. The first is the recurrent unicystic ameloblastoma. A tumor that recurs following a well-performed enucleation and curettage should probably be approached with the more aggressive resection. Second is the mural ameloblastoma. This variant of the unicystic ameloblastoma is probably more aggressive than the luminal and intraluminal variants of the unicystic ameloblastoma owing to the presence of tumor in the cyst wall and therefore closer to the surrounding bone. It seems logical to ap-

proach these tumors with a surgery similar to that for the solid or multicystic ameloblastoma. The final indication for resection of a unicystic ameloblastoma is in the management of very large tumors with significant expansion such that an enucleation and curettage surgery would effectively result in a resection of the involved jaw.

10.1.2.3   Peripheral ameloblastoma

The peripheral or extraosseous ameloblastoma is the rarest variant of the ameloblastoma. This tumor probably arises from rests of dental lamina or the basal epithelial cells of the surface epithelium and shows the same features of the intraosseous form of the tumor. Clinically, these tumors present as nonulcerated sessile or pedunculated gingival lesions. Most examples are < 1.5 cm and usually occur over a wide age range, with an average reported age of 52 years. Although these tumors do not infiltrate bone, they may be seen to "cup out" bone in the jaws.

The peripheral ameloblastoma is most appropriately treated with a wide local excision. When surgical margins are negative for tumor, cure is the likely consequence. Malignant transformation of a peripheral ameloblastoma is very rare.

10.2   Salivary Diseases

10.2.1   *Mucoceles and Ranulas*

Mucoceles are mostly due to extravasation of mucus from a salivary gland, although a few are true retention phenomena. The most common site is the lower lip, due to trauma (usually following an accidental bite in a child). Mucoceles are simple to treat and they should not recur if the underlying damaged minor salivary gland has been removed. Following a vertical incision through the mucosa over the mucocele, a number of minor salivary glands are usually identified. As it may be impossible to identify the damaged gland, all these minor glands should be removed before carefully suturing the mucosal incision.

Ranulas are large retention phenomena that occur in the floor of the mouth in relation to the sublingual gland. They may be large enough to elevate the tongue and interfere with speech and swallowing. Where dehiscence in the mylohyoid muscle occurs, the mucus can drain into the submandibular space as a "plunging ranula". The treatment of ranulas has been reviewed at length in a classic paper by

Catone. He concluded that definitive therapy was removal of the sublingual gland. Several large series have been reported comparing sublingual gland excision with so-called marsupialization, demonstrating 100% cure for gland excision and 43% to 63% cure for marsupialization.

Despite this evidence some authorities still plead the case for marsupialization or "marsupialization with packing," which they claim has a lower recurrence rate of 10% to 12%. We subscribe to the view that ranulas should be treated by sublingual gland excision.

An intraoral approach is made with an incision along the axis of the gland lateral to the ductal orifices. The submandibular duct is identified, either by dissection or following cannulation with a lacrimal probe. The gland is dissected in a subcapsular plane with meticulous hemostasis. At its posterior pole the lingual nerve is identified as it crosses the duct and is preserved. The sublingual gland is dissected from anteriorly, and the final excision is the posterior pole after visualizing the lingual nerve.

10.2.2   Pleomorphic Adenoma

Tumors of the salivary glands show a wide variety of pathologic types varying from benign to highly malignant. The pleomorphic adenoma is the most common benign salivary tumor at all sites. Approximately 80% of all pleomorphic adenomas (PSAs) occur in the parotid, and despite their slow growth they can become extremely large if neglected. This tumor is thought to arise from both salivary ducts and myoepithelial cells and is a true "mixed tumor". Because of its derivation, histologically, many different patterns can occur, from cellular, glandular, and myxoid types to cartilaginous and even ossified forms. These features can be seen in different areas of the same tumor, accounting for its name, *pleomorphic* (Greek for many forms). The important feature from a surgical standpoint is the presence of a "pseudo capsule", which contains outgrowths or pseudopodia of the tumor. Attempts at "enucleation" of the tumor from within its "capsule" will inevitably leave viable tumor cell nests and predispose the patient to multifocal recurrence. Some authorities believe that younger patients with pleomorphic adenomas have a higher chance of tumor recurrence and increased growth during pregnancy. Malignant change is rare and usually takes place in long-standing tumors, the most common type being carcinoma

ex pleomorphic adenoma. Prognosis will depend on the type of malignancy and involvement of the capsule. Rarely, malignant change in both elements of the pleomorphic adenoma (ductal and myoepithelial) will occur giving rise to the carcinosarcoma or true mixed malignant (biphasic) pleomorphic adenoma. On rare occasions, an apparently histologically benign tumor will metastasize into the so-called benign metastasizing pleomorphic adenoma.

Diagnostic imaging with computed tomography (CT) or magnetic resonance (MR) is desirable for superficial lobe tumors but is essential for suspected deep-lobe neoplasms, especially those with a parapharyngeal component. Since 80% of parotid tumors are benign and 80% of these are pleomorphic adenomas, a solitary mass in the parotid with no features of malignancy is most likely a PSA.

Open biopsy of such a mass is therefore contraindicated as this will rupture the "capsule" and "seed" the PSA, increasing the complexity of subsequent surgery and chances of recurrence.

Fine-needle aspiration biopsy (FNAB) for cytology is the preferred method of diagnosis. 6 Clinically only one-third of malignant tumors will have symptoms or signs of malignancy, such as pain, ulceration of skin, facial nerve palsy, or metastatic cervical nodes. Thus virtually all parotid tumors will initially be treated as benign unless FNAB shows definite malignancy or there is clinical evidence of malignancy.

The majority of tumors occur in the superficial lobe, and superficial lobectomy with preservation of the facial nerve has been the standard operation for many years. Recent minor modifications have included the use of a face-lift incision, the use of the superficial musculoaponeurotic system to prevent Frey's syndrome, the use of flaps or alloplasts to augment defects, and the suggestion that "capsular dissection" without the need to remove the entire superficial parotid may be sufficient. Superficial lobectomy is suitable for benign and low-grade malignant tumors, and even in high-grade malignancies only branches of the nerve that are actually infiltrated will be sacrificed. If the nerve or portions of it have to be resected, immediate grafting is recommended.

In deep-lobe tumors a total parotidectomy is performed, with the superficial lobe being dissected first to expose the nerve. Good margins with surrounding normal salivary gland tissue are more difficult to obtain on deep-lobe tumors, which tend to be large as they are often detected late.

In high-grade tumors, surrounding tissues such as skin, masseter, and mandible may require sacrifice, as dictated by the need to obtain clear margins. In these instances consideration should be given to neck dissection. Where clinically positive nodes are present, a modified radical neck dissection is usually the operation of choice. 11 Where the patient is N0 clinically, but at high risk for occult nodal disease, a selective neck dissection of levels I to IV or levels II to IV is indicated.

In high-grade tumors postoperative radiation therapy is usually indicated. Chemotherapy has not been shown to convey a survival benefit for these lesions.

10. 3 Premalignant Diseases

Premalignant diseases can be divided into that occurring as an isolated lesion or that associated with a condition. A precancerous lesion is defined as morphologically altered tissue in which the development of malignancy is more likely than with normal mucosa. A precancerous condition is a condition or generalized disease that does not necessarily alter the appearance of the mucosa but may be associated with a greater risk for the development of cancer. Precancerous lesions are broadly classified as leukoplakia and erythroplakia.

10. 3. 1 Leukoplakia

Leukoplakia is defined as a white patch or plaque that cannot be characterized clinically or ascribed to any other pathologic disease. Leukoplakia cannot be scraped or rubbed off and is therefore primarily a diagnosis of exclusion. Lesions caused by lichen planus, white sponge nevus, nicotine stomatitis, or other plaque-causing diseases do not qualify as leukoplakia. Leukoplakia is strictly a clinical diagnosis and does not imply any specific histologic diagnosis. Leukoplakia is generally asymptomatic and clinically appears as a white or off-white lesion that may be flat, slightly elevated, rugated, or smooth. It may be found as isolated or multifocal lesions and may change in morphology over time. More than 70% of the time leukoplakia occurs on two or more surfaces and has a strong male predilection. A more aggressive variant exists and is referred to as proliferative verrucous leukoplakia. The lower lip vermilion, buccal mucosa, and gingiva account for most oral cavity leukoplakia; however, lesions found on the tongue and floor of the

mouth account for most lesions exhibiting dysplasia or carcinoma. These relative frequencies change with different geographic locations and are based on local habits.

The only consistent histology found in all leukoplakia is the presence of hyperkeratosis. The underlying epithelium may range from normal to invasive carcinoma. The true etiology for the development of leukoplakia is unknown; however, several causative factors have been proposed. Tobacco use, whether smoked or smokeless, is most closely associated with the development of leukoplakia, and more than 70% of patients with leukoplakia are smokers. While several studies have shown elimination of tobacco use to be associated with resolution or decrease in the size of the lesion, others have shown poor improvement with its cessation.

Ultraviolet radiation to the lower lip is frequently observed in the development of lower lip vermilion leukoplakia. Individuals with chronic unprotected exposure to sunlight are at highest risk for development. These leukoplakia lesions are frequently associated with actinic cheilitis.

Trauma is also associated with the development of leukoplakic lesions. Ill fitting dentures, sharp edges on oral prostheses or teeth, or parafunctional oral habits with objects such as toothpicks can be associated with leukoplakia. Obvious traumatic lesions to the buccal mucosa such as the development of a linea alba are not considered leukoplakia.

The frequency of dysplasia and carcinoma within leukoplakia is most closely associated with the lesion's location and patient's habits. Waldron and Shafer in their study of 3,256 lesions submitted to their respective oral pathology departments as "leukoplakia" found that 43% of floor-of-mouth lesions and 24% of both tongue and lip lesions contained some degree of dysplasia or carcinoma. Several studies have also looked at malignant transformation over time and found it to vary from 0.13% to 17.5%. The results of these studies vary according to suspected causes of the leukoplakia (geographic habits) and the length of follow-up or time to biopsy of the lesion. The malignant transformation of these lesions has been studied extensively by Silverman and colleagues. They note that, while a definite rate of transformation cannot be stated, their 257 patients had a 17.5% transformation rate with an average follow-up time of 7.1 years. The second year of follow-up in their series exhibited the greatest rate of malignant transformation at 5%. If those lesions initially noted to be dysplastic on biopsy were followed, they had an even higher rate of malignant transformation, at 36.4%. Earlier studies by Silverman and colleagues found malignant transformation rates of 0.13% and 6%. The variability in transformation rates of most studies is attributed to differences in ethnicity, drinking alcohol and tobacco usage, location of the lesions, and duration of follow-up.

10.3.2   Erythroplakia

Erythroplakia is a red patch that cannot be scraped off or characterized clinically or ascribed to any other pathologic disease. Almost all true erythroplakia demonstrates dysplasia, carcinoma in situ, or invasive carcinoma. Shafer and Waldron's review of biopsies submitted under this clinical diagnosis revealed that 51% were invasive SCC, 40% were carcinoma in situ or severe dysplasia, and 9% were mild to moderate dysplasia. The most common sites of occurrence are the floor of the mouth and retromolar trigone. Lesions appear as bright red, are frequently "velvety" in appearance, and have a sharply demarcated border. The etiology of these lesions is unknown but thought to be the same as that for leukoplakia. Frequently these lesions are noted to be nonhomogeneous in appearance with adjacent or intralesional leukoplakia. When observed with this morphology, they are referred to as erythroleukoplakia or "speckled erythroplakia". These lesions also harbor an ominous potential as rates of malignant transformation have been noted of up to 23%.

10.3.3   Oral Submucous Fibrosis

Oral submucous fibrosis (OSF) is a precancerous condition seen predominantly in India and Southeast Asia. It is a chronic, progressive mucosal disorder most frequently associated with the habit of chewing betel quid; however, there is evidence that this lesion is multifactorial in nature with genetic, immunologic, nutritional, and autoimmune factors possibly involved. The condition is characterized by a mucosal rigidity that leads to trismus, odynophagia with spicy foods, and difficulty with speech and swallowing. Unlike tobacco pouch keratosis, OSF does not regress with the cessation of betel quid use. Longitudinal studies have shown a malignant transformation rate of 7.6% over a 17-year period.

10.3.4   Management of Premalignant Lesions

Leukoplakia is defined as a predominately white lesion of the oral mucosa that cannot be characterized as any other definable lesion. Worldwide estimates of its prevalence range from 1.5% to 2.6%. Lower socioeconomic status seems to be associated with higher prevalence. The potential for malignant transformation of oral leukoplakia to invasive squamous cell carcinoma is well recognized, and leukoplakia can be considered a precancerous lesion (i.e. "a morphologically altered tissue in which cancer is more likely to occur than in its apparent normal counterpart"). Estimated rates of transformation, however, vary widely. This most likely relates to the heterogeneity of the lesions included in most studies. While homogeneous white leukoplakia has a relatively low risk, erythroleukoplakia has a high incidence of associated dysplasia, carcinoma in situ, and frank carcinoma. In their often-quoted study of 257 patients followed for a mean of 8 years, Silverman and colleagues found transformation rates for leukoplakia to range from 6.5% for homogeneous lesions to 23.4% in erythroplasia. Lesions containing dysplasia had a transformation rate of 36.4%. The annual transformation rate in one population was less than 1%, which still demonstrated a 36-fold risk increase for squamous cell carcinoma in patients with oral leukoplakia over the population in general.

Predicting which lesions will ultimately transform is currently not possible. Given its asymptomatic nature, the sole indication for treatment of leukoplakia is an attempt to prevent subsequent malignant transformation. Treatment modalities include excision, ablation, and chemoprevention. Unfortunately no treatment modality has been shown to prevent subsequent development of squamous cell carcinoma.

The first Cochrane review on therapy for leukoplakia did not find any reliable therapy to prevent the transformation of leukoplakia to oral squamous cell carcinoma. Also, there were no effective preventive measures to halt the development of oral leukoplakia. No surgical procedures were included in this review because of the lack of randomized clinical trials evaluating surgical excision. Chemopreventive agents including retinoids, beta carotene, green tea, and bleomycin were evaluated. Retinoids held the most promise and were associated with resolution of lesions. The ultimate goal remains prevention of subsequent malignant transformation, and unfortunately none of the agents demonstrated this reliably. In addition associated side effects were problematic.

Surgical excision remains an alternative for dealing with worrisome lesions. CO_2 laser excision has been used to treat widespread superficial lesions in an attempt to limit scarring and morbidity associated with large excisions. Laser ablation allows the destruction of large superficial lesions. It does not provide a histologic specimen, however, and biopsies from any areas of ulceration or erythroplasia are probably indicated prior to ablation. Unfortunately recurrence following laser excision or ablation is not uncommon, and it does not necessarily prevent malignant transformation.

Given the high rates of multiple lesions and their propensity to recur, photodynamic therapy (PDT) is gaining popularity as a potential method for dealing with multiple diffuse lesions. PDT relies on a complex interaction of a photosensitizing agent, which is preferentially concentrated in abnormal tissue, with light of various wavelengths, depending on the photosensitizer, to create necrosis through a nonthermal reaction. Tissue necrosis is mediated through the creation of singlet oxygen, a highly reactive species that induces cellular damage through several mechanisms. Advantages of PDT include minimal damage to surrounding tissues and no cumulative damage, which theoretically allows unlimited treatments. Given the propensity for these patients to develop multiple lesions, this is an important advantage over excision or ablation using traditional methods. Disadvantages include marked photosensitivity, especially with regard to sun exposure, for variable lengths of time after the administration of the agent. Areas treated undergo healing through mucosalization with minimal or no scarring. Although a complete review of PDT is beyond the scope of this chapter, excellent reviews are available.

PDT has been used with some success in the endoscopic treatment of dysplastic Barrett's esophagitis to prevent its transformation to adenocarcinoma. Similarly attempts have been made to treat diffuse oral leukoplakia with PDT with some success. In addition to its role in the management of leukoplakia, initial trials of PDT applied to invasive squamous cell carcinoma of selected sites in the head and neck are being reported. Copper and colleagues reported on 25 patients with T1 and T2 lesions of the oral cavity and oropharynx treated with PDT. Complete remission was noted in 86% of lesions. Recurrences were salvaged with conventional therapy. In addition to its application to mucosal lesions, interstitial delivery of light may allow treatment of more deeply situated tumors. Although results are promising, PDT for leukoplakia and oral cavity cancers remains investigational, and its role in the management of leukoplakia and squamous cell cancers of the head and neck awaits clarification.

10.4 Oral Cancer

Mortality rates remain high despite some advances in locoregional control. There will be approximately 200,000 deaths worldwide. Most patients will present for diagnosis with either regional or distant disease. A review of trends in 5-year relative survival rates over the past three decades has shown a statistical difference between the time periods of 1974 to 1976 and 1992 to 1996 (54% vs. 59%). Approximately 85% to 95% of all oral cancer is squamous cell carcinoma (SCC). However, multiple other malignant lesions can be found in the oral cavity such as sarcoma, minor salivary gland tumors, mucosal melanoma, lymphoma, or metastatic disease from nearly any site in the body.

10.4.1 Risk Factors for SCC of the Oral Cavity

The etiology of SCC of the oral cavity has been studied extensively. Numerous risk factors have been suggested as etiologic agents for the development of these malignancies. While no single causative agent can be attributed to the development of all oral cancers, several carcinogens have been identified, and of those tobacco and alcohol appear to have the greatest impact on malignancy development. Both extrinsic and intrinsic factors likely play a role in the development of SCC of the oral cavity.

The risk of oral cancer associated with tobacco use is noted to be 2 to 12 times higher than in the nonsmoking population, and 90% of individuals with oral cancer will have a smoking history. The combination of various carcinogens within tobacco, combined with the heat, may lead to a variable number of genetic mutations in the epithelium of the upper aerodigestive tract. At some point these continued mutations, coupled with the patients' own inherent genetic susceptibility, expressed in the hetero- or homogeneity of certain tumor suppressor genes or oncogenes (*TP53*, *c-myc*), may lead to the development of a cell line capable of unregulated growth.

Alcohol in itself is not a recognized initiator in the development of oral SCC. However, the role of alcohol as a promoter in the development of oral cancer when coupled with the use of smoking tobacco has been shown. This may be related to the effects of contaminants in alcohol and its ability to solubilize carcinogens and enhance their penetration into oral mucosa.

A possible viral etiology has been demonstrated in oral cancers, especially by the human papilloma virus (HPV). The HPV subtypes 16 and 18, similar to those causing cervical cancer, have been implicated. Smith and colleagues showed that when individuals in his study had other risk factors adjusted, such as smoking, alcohol, and age, the presence of HPV in the oral cavity was associated with a 3. 7 times greater chance of cancer development than in the noninfected individual. Other authors have noted a unique subset of characteristics in individuals that may develop SCC as a result of HPV infection, showing less association with tobacco or alcohol abuse, frequently involving the tonsils, and having an improved prognosis.

The study of the tumor biology of SCC has exploded in the past decade. The accepted molecular theory concerning genetic alterations of SCC is that of a "multihit" tumorigenesis ultimately leading to unregulated cell growth and function. It is thought that multiple exogenous insults (tobacco, alcohol, viral) can lead to activation of oncogenes or inactivation of tumor suppressor genes. Oncogene dysregulation leads to a gain of function alteration, and transforming growth factor alpha (TGF-α) and eukaryotic initiation factor 4E (eIF4E) are two examples of well-studied genes that have proven upregulation in SCC. Loss of tumor suppressor gene function requires loss of both normal alleles, which leads to the inactivation of the critical function of that gene. The most studied of the tumor suppressor genes are *TP53* and *P16*. No single gene alteration is responsible for carcinogenesis, but rather a host of altered genes contribute. Attempts have been made to use genes and their products to identify oncologically safe margins operatively with minimal success. Gene therapy trials that target these specific genes hold better promise.

10. 4. 2   Staging

The TNM system devised by the AJCC is designed to stratify cancer patients into different stages based on the characteristics of the primary tumor (T), regional lymph node metastasis (N), and distant metastasis (M). It is an attempt to help guide treatment and estimate patients' 5-year survivability. *T* refers to the primary lesion and is graded on greatest dimension and presence of adjacent tissue infiltration. *N* refers to regional lymph node involvement and is graded on the presence of nodes, greatest dimension, and side of involvement in relation to the primary tumor. *M* grades distant metastasis and is based simply on its presence (M1) or absence (M0). The AJCC staging system is designed for clinical use; however, the patient may be restaged based on final pathology after resection and designated with a *p* prefix (pTNM) or at autopsy with an *a* (aTNM). If synchronous tumors are found at presentation, the higher stage tumor should be used for stage designation, and an *m* suffix may be used to denote the multiple primary tumors (TmNM).

10. 4. 3   Diagnosis

A thorough clinical examination is the first line of defense in the detection of oral cancer. Prognosis is directly dependent on the tumor stage at diagnosis. Nearly one-half of all oral cancers are not detected until they are in advanced stages. This delay may be because symptoms may not develop until later in the disease process or the socioeconomic group most likely to develop oral cancer is unable to seek treatment until it has reached an advanced stage. A study by Holmes and colleagues showed that detection of oral and oropharyngeal SCC during non-symptom-driven examinations was associated with a lower stage at diagnosis.

Once a clinically suspicious lesion is identified in the oral cavity, tissue diagnosis must be obtained prior to rendering any treatment. This biopsy can usually be done in an office setting or rarely under general anesthesia with panendoscopy if the lesion is difficult to access and patient tolerance is low. The traditional biopsy, whether incisional or excisional (for small lesions), is the gold standard. It should be emphasized that an accurate dimension of the lesion should be acquired prior to biopsy in order to properly stage the lesion. When faced with a large lesion, it is best to take several biopsies from different sites in an attempt to decrease any sampling error that might be read as dysplasia, necrosis, or inflammation.

Management of the regional lymphatics is a consideration in any cancer. The ability of a cancer to metastasize most commonly manifests itself by growth of cancer in lymph nodes. Evaluation of the neck for cervical metastases remains a critical component of the evaluation of the patient with oral cavity cancer. Manual palpation is regarded as the first step in this process and is usually accomplished before biopsy to avoid postbiopsy inflammatory nodal enlargement. In most necks a lymph node must be at least 1 cm in diameter to be palpable. The accuracy and reliability of palpation is low, with an overall error of approximately 30% in several studies. Imaging modalities including CT, MRI, ultrasonography, and positron emission tomography (PET) have become increasingly important in the evaluation for cervical metastases and in guiding therapy.

A CT scan with contrast from the skull base to clavicles has become the most common imaging modality used for detection of cervical metastases. Specific criteria for nodal metastases, including node size greater than 1 cm (except the jugulodigastric node, which must be greater than 1.5 cm), central necrosis, and morphology (round instead of oval) have increased sensitivity to over 90%. MRI neck evaluation has gained popularity in recent years, and is typically used if the primary site is being imaged with MRI, such as for a tongue cancer. CT and MRI, in that order, are the most widely used imaging modalities for detection of occult metastases.

The characteristics of the primary tumor may also predict metastases. Spiro and colleagues demonstrated that depth of invasion in tongue cancer was a reliable predictor of lymph node metastases in cancer of the oral tongue. They found that cancers with 2 to 8 mm depth of invasion had a significantly higher rate of lymph node metastases than those with invasion of less than 2 mm (25.7% vs. 7.5%). Depth of invasion greater than 8 mm was associated with a 41% rate of occult metastasis. Tumor thickness less than 2 mm has been associated with a 13% incidence of lymph node metastases and 3% would ultimately succumb to their disease, whereas greater than 9 mm of invasion was associated with a 65% incidence of lymph node metastases and 35% would die of their disease. O-charoenrat and colleagues also demonstrated an increased risk of cervical metastasis in tongue cancers with a depth of invasion greater than 5 mm, and correlated this with poor outcome even in early stage (I and II) tongue

cancers. Similar results were reported by Kurokawa and colleagues, who found that depth greater than 4 mm was associated with an increased risk for development of late cervical metastases in patients with moderately differentiated squamous cell cancers of the tongue, and diminished overall survival. This has led to recommendations that even in the absence of evidence of lymph node metastases, the neck should receive elective treatment (either elective neck dissection or irradiation) for thicker primary tumors. Other investigators have suggested that depth of invasion be added to the staging of oral squamous cell carcinomas. Aside from depth, clinicians have looked at other characteristics such as DNA aneuploidy and histologic grade. At this time applications of this technology have not been adopted in the routine clinical setting.

Two additional imaging modalities used for evaluating nodal metastases deserve mention. Ultrasonography and PET with fluorodeoxyglucose are gaining in popularity for initial staging and follow-up staging of patients with head and neck cancer. Ultrasonography criteria for malignant changes include nodal size and changes in echogenicity, central necrosis that will lead to an echogenic hilum, and a hypoechogenic periphery. Its ability to improve on manual palpation of cervical lymphadenopathy has led to its increased use. It can also help to evaluate carotid or jugular invasion. When performed by an experienced clinician and combined with aspiration cytology, ultrasonography is very accurate.

Recently PET has become increasingly popular in the staging and follow-up of patients with head and neck squamous cell carcinoma. By identifying areas of high glucose uptake, PET scans allow clinicians to identify potential metastases in the preoperative work-up. Presence of distant metastases may influence the choice of initial treatment. The role of PET scans in the evaluation of occult cervical metastases is limited by the need for at least 5 to 10 mm3 of tumor for detection. Their role in the work-up of patients with cervical metastases and unknown primaries continues to be explored. PET is also used to examine patients who have undergone chemoradiotherapy for recurrent disease. These patients are notorious for their difficulty in examination secondary to extensive changes in the soft tissue. It is recommended that at least 3 months pass prior to obtaining a PET scan because of the persistent inflammation associated with radiation and the tumoricidal effects that persist after radiation is completed. It should also be remembered that current technology requires that a focus of squamous cell carcinoma be several millimeters to be detected. In the past it was stated that distant metastases were a late finding in head and neck cancer patients and most patients succumbed to locoregional disease. It was felt that less than 1% of head and neck cancer patients had distant disease at presentation. As the use of PET scanning in the initial evaluation of patients with oral cavity cancers becomes more widespread, detection of distant metastases at the initial evaluation may become more common. One result of these improvements in detection of distant disease is **stage migration.** In other words, as our ability to detect distant disease improves, more patients are staged higher. This does not mean that patients are being diagnosed later in the course of their disease than in the past but simply that our diagnostic abilities have improved.

10. 4. 4   Treatment

Once the initial evaluation, data collection, and staging are complete, a discussion regarding treatment is undertaken. The clinician and the patient are faced with deciding which treatment modality or combination offers not only the best chance for cure, but also quality of life. Quality-of-life issues are becoming increasingly important in treatment planning. Despite media hyperbole on cancer treatment "breakthroughs," cancer treatment still falls into three basic categories: surgery, radiation, or chemotherapy, or some combination thereof. Choosing the appropriate treatment relies on many factors, including the patient's medical condition as well as the modalities available to the clinician. Certain therapeutic modalities, such as neutron beam radiotherapy, may hold promise for certain tumors, but are limited in their availability. Although each will be discussed separately in the upcoming sections, most patients will ultimately receive more than one form of treatment.

The oral tongue, that portion anterior to the circumvallate papillae, is the most common location for intraoral squamous cell carcinomas. They typically present as painless indurated ulcerations. If pain is present it is usually due to secondary infection. The behavior and treatment of oral tongue cancers is sufficiently different than that of posterior tongue lesions (oropharyngeal tongue or tongue

base) to allow clinicians to determine the epicenter of the tumor and classify it correctly. This may be challenging in the case of larger cancers. The oral tongue poses significant challenges to clinicians. Seemingly small lesions can metastasize early and recur after treatment. Control rates for small lesions of the tongue (60% to 80%) are poorer than those of similar size in other oral cavity subsites. There are minimal barriers in the tongue to tumor invasion, and there is frequent invasion into adjacent or deeper structures at presentation. Although more commonly associated with oropharyngeal primary cancers, referred otalgia is not uncommon for cancers of the oral tongue, and limitation of tongue mobility with resultant dysarthria is associated with invasion of the deeper musculature. MRI can be useful in evaluating the depth of invasion. Treatment of tongue lesions should be aggressive, and strong consideration for elective treatment of the neck should be given in all cases except for the most superficial lesions (<2 mm). Up to 10% to 12% of tongue cancers with metastases to the neck can demonstrate "skip" metastases to level IV. Consideration should be given to extending the neck dissection to include level IV. Postoperative radiation should be considered in situations where multiple frozen-section specimens were sent before obtaining clear margins, perineural invasion, microvascular or microlymphatic invasion, or other worrisome findings that are present.

Smaller superficial tumors are amenable to wide local excision and reconstruction via primary closure, split-thickness skin grafting, or healing by secondary intention. Larger tumors are reconstructed with vascularized tissue transfer, and mandibulectomy may be needed for adequate access to large or posterior lesions. Radial forearm or lateral arm microvascular free flaps allow excellent mobility and little bulk. Unilateral or bilateral pedicled nasolabial flaps can occasionally be used for anterior tongue lesions. Large oral tongue cancers that cross the midline present the surgeon with a difficult choice. If resection is chosen it is often better to tailor the radial forearm flap smaller than the resected area to allow the remaining tongue musculature less bulk to move during excursions. Near total glossectomy (resection of the oral tongue with only tongue base remaining) almost always results in high morbidity and is associated with a high incidence of aspiration that may ultimately require laryngectomy for aspiration control. Treatment with external beam radiation alone is associated with unacceptable failure rates. In this setting consideration should be given to organ-sparing protocols with concomitant chemoradiation therapy if surgery will be associated with unacceptable morbidity. Brachytherapy combined with external beam radiation is the treatment of choice at some centers. Technical expertise is required, and most patients require tracheotomy for airway control. Tongue base tumors, although actually an oropharyngeal subsite and not considered an oral subsite, are discussed here for completeness.

The tongue base allows tumors to grow silently, and diagnosis at an early stage is the exception rather than the rule. Most small (T1 and some T2) lesions should be treated with combined therapy, typically surgery plus radiation treatment. Larger tumors are typically treated with an organ-sparing approach using chemoradiation therapy or external beam therapy, sometimes combined with brachytherapy. Results with external beam alone have been disappointing. Reconstruction of smaller posterior tongue defects is best accomplished by radial forearm or lateral arm flaps, if primary closure or healing by secondary intention is inappropriate. Larger excisions (75% to total) typically are reconstructed with a free rectus flap.

Most treatment failures of the oral tongue involve locoregional recurrence. Second primary cancer rates are high (30%) and this also contributes to treatment failure and death. Three-year survival for T1 and T2 lesions is 70% to 80%, but this decreases to 15% to 30% in patients with lymph node metastases. Some clinicians have reported that tongue squamous cell carcinoma arising in young patients may represent a more aggressive subset and warrant more aggressive therap. Overall survival for younger patients is actually similar to those of older patients with the same stage because of their lack of intercurrent illnesses. It was found, however, that oral tongue cancers in younger women did behave more aggressively and were associated with higher recurrence rates. This subset may warrant more aggressive initial therapy.

Gingival squamous cell cancers represent a unique subset in oral cavity cancers that arise on the attached gingiva and that should be differentiated from those that arise on the unattached mucosa of the alveolus. Occult neck metastasis is rare, and elective treatment of the neck is not necessary in smaller lesions. Larger lesions may require partial maxillectomy, or marginal or segmental mandibulectomy, if bone invasion is suspected. Indications and variations on mandibulectomy are discussed below. In general control rates are excellent for gingival primary cancers if treated with adequate margins.

Alveolar cancer arises from the unattached mucosa of the alveolar ridge and has a different clinical behavior than gingival carcinomas. It requires more aggressive therapy and more extensive resection of bone.

Most anterior and some posterior maxillectomies for alveolar and gingival squamous cells can be accomplished via a transoral approach using techniques of orthognathic surgery. The pterygoid plates require removal only if there is evidence of invasion through the posterior maxilla. Posterior extension may indicate the need for a transfacial (Weber-Fergusson) approach for adequate exposure. Reconstruction of maxillary defects can be accomplished with local flaps, such as the temporoparietal fascial or temporalis muscle flap, or free-flap reconstruction. The complex nature of maxillary defects and the bulk of some of the flaps, however, often leave a less-than-satisfactory result. Prosthetic obturation of the defect offers several advantages, including a simpler operation, easier early detection of recurrence, and replacement of teeth.

Most maxillary alveolus and gingival squamous cells that invade the sinus involve the infrastructure lying below Ohngren's line, an artificial line that runs from the medial canthus to the angle of the mandible and separates the maxillary sinus into an infra- and supra-structure. Defects arising from cancers resected below this line are easily reconstructed with obturators. Cancers that require true total maxillectomy (resection of one of the paired maxillas, including the orbital floor) tend to require flap reconstruction. If dura mater is exposed as part of a skull base resection, flap coverage is advisable.

Overall 5-year survival for alveolar ridge carcinoma is 50% to 65% for both the upper and lower alveolar ridge. Poor outcome is associated with advanced stage, perineural spread, and positive margins. Adjunctive radiation is recommended if nodal metastases, perineural spread, or positive margins are present.

10.4.5   Recurrence and Follow-up Surveillance

In 1984, Vikram and colleagues published a series of reports that discussed patterns of failure in patients treated with multimodality therapy for head and neck cancer. This classic series of articles outlined failure characteristics at the local site, neck, distant sites, as well as development of second malignant neoplasms in patients treated at Memorial Sloan-Kettering Cancer Center, USA. Ninety percent of patients who will suffer a recurrence of oral cavity cancer will do so in the first 2 years. For this reason patients are placed in a structured follow-up. Stage at recurrence is the most important predictor of survival, with stage I at recurrence associated with a median survival of 24. 3 months and a disease-free survival at 2 years of 73%, whereas stage IV recurrence was associated with a median survival of 9. 3 months and a 2-year disease free survival of 22%. Follow-up protocols vary widely and are intended to detect recurrences early. De Visscher and Manni suggested the following:

(1) Every 2 months for year 1.
(2) Every 3 months for year 2.
(3) Every 4 months for year 3.
(4) Every 6 months for years 4 and 5.
(5) Then yearly.

Despite this and other suggested follow-up protocols, the follow-up schedule must be tailored to the individual patient and must take into account the patient's likelihood of having a recurrence, possible continuation of smoking or other habits, ability to travel and keep appointments, and the potential availability of local medical or dental care that might assist in follow-up surveillance. Follow-up appointments include an update of patient history and review of systems as well as clinical examination for recurrence or detection of new primaries. Questions raised by physical examination should prompt an appropriate imaging study, rebiopsy, or examination under anesthesia. Caution should be used, however, in performing biopsies in patients who have received intensive multimodality therapy, such as RAD-PLAT, brachytherapy, or hyperfractionated radiation schedules combined with chemotherapy. Extensive biopsy wounds are notorious for slow healing and can lead to chronic wounds.

Appropriate imaging, including a baseline CT or MRI at the completion of multimodality therapy, is invaluable. The role of PET scanning in follow-up continues to evolve.

Failure at the primary cancer site will ultimately occur in approximately 20% of patients, and regional recurrence in the neck will occur in 10%. Death

from distant metastases is rare, occurring in only about 1% to 4% of cases in which locoregional control is maintained. An unfortunate consequence of improved control at the primary cancer site with multimodality therapy is an increasing incidence of distant metastases. In addition to recurrences, prospective studies have demonstrated that second primary cancers develop at a rate of 4% to 7% annually in patients who have had a head and neck squamous cancer. Second primary cancers are the leading cause of death among patients who have undergone treatment for early stage oral cancers.

The ability of a cancer to metastasize depends on the development of a series of genetic mutations, allowing for cells to disseminate from the primary tumor, arrest in the microcirculation, extravagate, infiltrate into stroma, and survive and proliferate as a new colony. Surveillance for distant metastase therefore becomes an important component of the follow-up evaluation. The lungs are the most common site for distant metastases, followed by the liver and bone. Yearly or biannual chest radiographs allow for detection of lung metastases, the most common distant site metastasized for oral cavity cancer, and primary lung cancers, which are not uncommon in the population at risk for oral cancer. Given the current unavailability of an effective treatment regimen, however, some authors have questioned the use of annual or semiannual chest radiographs. PET scanning may prove to be a more valuable alternative for detection of distant disease. Yearly lab work to include liver function studies is also recommended. In patients who have received radiation as part of their treatment, periodic thyroid function tests are helpful, as many will ultimately become hypothyroid with attendant fatigue and decreased wound healing ability.

Collins stated that patients with head and neck cancer are probably never cured, and that it is better to consider that the host-tumor relationship has been durably altered in favor of the host. It is important to realize that approximately one-third of patients with presumed localized disease will relapse and die of cancer. In advanced head and neck squamous cell carcinoma 20% to 30% will survive, 40% to 60% of patients will suffer locoregional recurrence, and 20% to 30% will succumb to distant metastases. Hence the majority of treatment failures remain recurrence of locoregional disease. Patients with recurrent disease are restaged, which requires a similar evaluation as the original. Panendoscopy and examination under anesthesia take on greater importance when a clinician is faced with examination of tissue scarred and distorted by previous surgery and radiation. Distant metastases should be ruled out to the extent possible prior to deciding on aggressive retreatment. It the patient does have recurrence that is confined to the locoregional area, treatment decisions are limited by previous therapy. Reirradiation protocols exist but are accompanied by significant morbidity. Intensive reirradiation and chemotherapy protocols are being investigated and show some promise. The morbidity of such treatments is significant, and their use should be restricted to clinical trials at this time. Surgical salvage remains the primary option, but the extent of salvage surgery must be considerably broader than might initially be considered. Goodwin reported on the outcome of salvage surgery for recurrent head and neck cancers, and found benefit in stages I and II. Success was limited in more advanced disease. Clearly defined goals should be established between surgeon and patient for salvage surgery. Is the operation for cure or palliation? Palliative surgery should be undertaken very cautiously as surgical complications may greatly overshadow the palliative goals. Patients and their families must have realistic expectations as well as understand that there is no benefit from repeated surgical intervention for recalcitrant cancer.

Patients with inoperable cancer pose a unique challenge to the clinician. As cure is no longer a realistic option, treatment modalities to prolong life and improve quality of life assume a higher priority. Pain control becomes a significant issue in patients with recurrent head and neck cancer. Long-acting sustained release formulations such as transdermal narcotic patches combined with short-acting narcotics for breakthrough pain are typically required. Rhizotomy is an option for intractable pain. Pain control can be a goal of palliative chemotherapy or radiotherapy. Novel methods for the targeted delivery of chemotherapeutic agents into the tumor are under development. A combination of cisplatin and epinephrine gel injected into recurrent tumors demonstrated significant palliation without significant side effects in most. Wound management becomes an important issue, and dealing with large malodorous wounds can be taxing on patients and families. Patients presenting with advanced head and neck cancer will typically survive 6 to 12 months without treat-

ment, and patients with end-stage head and neck cancer will have a median survival of 101 days.

There is a natural tendency for clinicians to avoid the dying patient. There is a reluctance to face a disease whose biology has resisted their best efforts and whose treatment has left patients debilitated and frequently deformed. While family members and clinicians are discussing further treatment options, patients are frequently simply concerned with pain control and the effects of massive doses of narcotics on bowel function. Frank, thoughtful discussions must be held with the patients and their families regarding end-of-life issues and will help surgeons deal with these very real concerns. Hospice provides an excellent resource, and once enrolled most families are appreciative of the support offered by these professionals in end-of-life care.

In this era of improved treatment modalities for local and regional disease, clinicians are finding that factors unrelated to the primary cancer and beyond their control are influencing survival. It is becoming increasingly evident that factors affecting outcome in oral cancer patients are multiple and may relate more to patient characteristics than the cancer itself or the treatment they receive. Researchers are finding that genetic factors of the primary cancer have an impact on the response of the particular tumor to any treatment. High expression of epidermal growth factor receptors is associated with poor outcome, and may indicate the need for more intensive multimodality therapy. Alterations in *TP*53 have been associated with recurrence in squamous cell cancer of the head and neck that was refractory to radiation treatment. Future treatments may include restoration of *TP*53 function.

Importantly studies are also demonstrating that comorbidities and performance status predict survival independent of stage at diagnosis. Performance status has been shown to be a predictor of survival independent of tumor, regional nodes, and metastasis (TNM) stage. Many head and neck cancer patients suffer other medical problems related to tobacco and alcohol use, and these can result in decreased overall survival despite cancer specific survival. Ribeiro and colleagues found that daily alcohol consumption, smoking, poor body mass index, and other comorbidities had an independent impact on prognosis. As discussed earlier there may indeed be a more aggressive form of squamous cell carcinoma that affects younger patients, but data from the

National Cancer Data Base indicate that younger patients have a survival advantage that is most likely related to their lack of comorbidities. Frequently 5- and 10- year survival curves are impacted more by these comorbidities than the tumor characteristics recorded in the TNM system. The TNM staging system will continue to undergo revisions to enhance its use.

■ Summary

The presentation of maxillofacial diseases is earlier than diseases from other regions of the body, and the early diagonsis of these diseases is not so easy because of the complexity of the maxillofacial pathology. The present chapter overviewed the most common maxillofacial diseases in each type of tissues with the hope to be benefit of the clinical early diagnosis and early treatment.

■ Questions

1. The clinical and pathological characteristics of pleomorphic adenoma of parotid?

2. The special treatment considerations of oral cancer based on site?

(**Zhengxue Han**　韩正学)

References

[1] Atula S, Grenman R, Laippala P, et al. Cancer of the tongue in patients younger than 40years. A distinct entity? Arch Otolaryngol Head Neck Surg, 1996, 122: 1313-1319.

[2] Baurmash HD. Mucoceles and ranulas. J Oral Maxillofac Surg, 2003, 61:369-378.

[3] Crysdale WS, Mandelsohn JD, Conley S. Ranulasmucocoeles of the oral cavity experience in 26 children. Laryngoscope, 1988, 98:296-298.

[4] Catone GA. Sublingual gland mucous escape. Pseudocysts of the oro-cervical region. Atlas Oral Maxillofac Surg Clin N Am, 1995, 7:431-477.

[5] DeVita VT, Hellman S, Rosenberg SA. Cancer: principles and practices of oncology. Philadelphia (PA): JB Lippincott Co. , 1993.

[6] Greene FL, Page DL, Fleming ID, et al. AJCC cancer staging manual. 6th ed. New York: Springer-Verlag, 2002.

[7] Kramer IRH, Pindborg JJ, Shear M. The WHO histological typing of odontogenic tumours. A commentary on the second edition. Cancer, 1992, 70:2988-2994.

[8] Neville BW, Damm DD, Allen CM, et al. Oral and maxillofacial pathology. Philadelphia: WB Saunders, 2002.

[9] Ord RA. Surgical management of parotid tumors. Atlas Oral Maxillofac Surg Clin N Am, 1995, 7:529-564.

[10] Pogrel MA, Jordan RCK. Marsupialization as a definitive treatment for odontogenic keratocysts. Chicago: American Association of Oral and Maxillofacial Surgeons, 2002.

[11] Regezi JA, Sciubba JJ, Jordan RCK. Oral pathology. Clinical pathologic correlations. St. Louis: WB Saunders, 2003.

[12] Myers EN, Suen JY. Cancer of the head and neck. 2nd ed. New York: Churchill Livingstone, 1987.

[13] Williams T. The ameloblastoma: a review of the literature. Selected readings in oral and maxillofacial surgery. Vol 2. San Francisco: The Guild for Scientific Advancement in Oral and Maxillofacial Surgery, 1991: 1-17.

[14] Yoshimura Y, Obara S, Kondoh T, et al. A comparison of three methods used for the treatment of ranula. J Oral Maxillofac Surg, 1995, 53:280-282.

Chapter 11

Geriatric Dentistry

▪ Objectives

The objective of the chapter is to provide a comprehensive review of the processes of aging and their relevance to the delivery or dental health care. Its target audiences are undergraduate and postgraduate students as well as practicing clinicians.

▪ Key Concepts

Dentistry for the elderly: For those who have not reached pensionable age, the elderly is anyone over 60. Others suggest that it is >65 yrs of age. Rather than arbitrary cut-offs, biological age should be considered.

Age changes are defined as an alteration in the form or function of a tissue or organ as a result of biological activity associated with a minor disturbance of normal cellular turnover.

▪ Introduction

This search is given extra emphasis by the dramatic increase in the proportions of older people in the populations of all countries. This trend is expected to continue, with the result that the elderly as a segment of society with special abilities as well as special needs, will become increasingly prominent.

The new generations of elderly will be better educated and more demanding of social and health services than past generations. Many will retain their natural teeth. These changes in health status, in attitude and behavior, will have a significant impact on oral health needs, creating new challenges for the dental profession.

The prevention and treatment of oral and dental diseases require a thorough knowledge of the biological variables influencing disease patterns in the aging patient. The relationship between oral and general health and the effects of chronic ailments and diseases on the ability of the older patient to accept treatment must be understood if dental health care is to have a reasonable chance of success. Dentist of tomorrow will need a broader range of knowledge, clinical skills, and human understanding to recognize and treat the oral health problems of their older patients. Cognizant of these needs, special courses and programs in dentistry for the elderly are being included in many undergraduate and graduate dental school curricula.

11. 1   Changes in the Oral Cavity with Aging

The gradual changes taking in the dental tissues after the teeth fully formed are referred to as age changes. The teeth are considered fully formed when the root apices have been completed, that is, approximately 6 months after a permanent tooth has reached occlusion.

Most tissues have a physiological turnover of their components. Epithelium replaces itself within days or weeks. Similar destruction and reconstruction occurs in connective tissue. The rate of turnover varies from tissue to tissue and depends on a number of local and systemic factors, including age. The growth factors that regulate cell proliferation have been characterized as peptides and proteins, and several types have been identified. Inhibitory or controlling substances, referred to as chalones, are also normally present and are specific to the various cell lines.

Some tissues are notable because they do not exhibit any turnover, for example, specialized cells such as those of the nervous system. Tooth enamel is also a tissue in which essentially no biological activity takes place after it is formed. In fact, in the proper sense of the term, enamel is more a material than a tissue, and its reactivity is limited to physicochemical processes. A limited turnover based on cellular activity is believed to occur in dentin and cementum. The pulp and especially the periodontal ligament, on the other hand, are examples of tissues in which the turnover is high.

Age changes are considered to be a result of biological activities and somehow tie up with minor disturbances in the normal turnover processes. Thus, the age changes are slow or non-existent in tissues that do not exhibit biological reactivity. Deviations from the normal biological activity may result in premature aging, that is, in tissue changes resembling those noted as age changes under normal conditions.

11. 1. 1   Changes in the Teeth with Aging

It is often difficult of impossible to differentiate between physiological age changes and the pathological changes that affect the teeth. Even erupted intact teeth are subjected to changes as a result of function. Strictly speaking, age changes should, therefore, possibly be limited to those that are found in unerupted teeth in adults of old individuals. However, impacted teeth are not normal per second. Thus, age changes in teeth cannot be considered in the strict sense of the term, but rather as frequently occurring changes found in functional, intact teeth from older individuals.

The teeth change in form and color with age. The tooth form is affected by wear and attrition. This process starts at an early age, for example, the loss of the incisal protuberances seen just after eruption. Apart from the occlusal, incisal and interproximal wear, a loss of structural details on the enamel surface is also noted over time. The perichymate and imbrication lines are lost, giving the enamel surface a flat appearance with less detail than in newly erupted teeth.

The altered surface structure gives the teeth in older individuals a different pattern of light reflection than that of young teeth. This feature causes a change in the observed color. Changes in the dentin, both in quantity (thickness) and quality (type of changes induced), also result in a gradual alteration in color with age. As the dentin contributes to the yellow shading of teeth, yellowing and a general loss of translucency are common age changes or teeth. Pigmentation of anatomical defects, corrosion products and inadequate oral hygiene may also change the tooth color.

Enamel

All changes in enamel are based on ion exchange mechanisms. It is generally accepted that enamel becomes less permeable and possibly more brittle with age, but little exact information appears to be available to substantiate these views. Bhussry and Hess reported no significant differences in the density of enamel as a function of age. However, the nitrogen content showed an increase with age. Their data indicated a constant nitrogen content of sound enamel in up to 30-year-old teeth. It then remains at a higher but constant level in teeth 30 to 60 years old. The last age group (61 – 70 years) showed a further increase. No explanation could be offered to account for the increase in organic material, but in appears feasible that the filling in of cracks in the enamel by organic material (acquired lamellae) may explain these findings.

Studies on the composition of surface and sub-surface (bulk) enamel have clearly demonstrated differences in chemistry between the two: for example, in fluoride content. The crystals in surface enamel are also much thicker than those in the bulk of the enamel. This difference in crystal size is not found in unerupted teeth. Experimentally exposed subsurface enamel has been shown to take on the characteristic of surface enamel fairly rapidly. The available data, therefore, indicate that the special properties of surface enamel are acquired.

Some of the acquired properties of surface enamel are slowly built up during life, such as the fluoride content. These changes in surface content may therefore be considered age changes. However, they are not due to aging per se, and they are not permanent because they are affected by attrition, abrasion and erosion. Caries also alters the chemistry of the surface enamel.

Cementum

Cementum may be resorbed and new cementum may form both locally in resorption defects and more generally over the root, especially in the apical half, to compensate for tooth wear during function. The susceptibility to resorption and the number of resorption areas increase with age, increased formation of cementum leads to a lack of nutrition of the cementocytes; they degenerate, and empty lacunae are often found in the deep layers of the cementum. These changes may be looked on as indirect age changes: processes that result in the changes occur as a result of alteration that is age-dependent per se. The composition of cementum has also been reported to change with age: for example, the fluoride and magnesium content.

Gingival recession is common in old individuals. The cervical acellular cementum, therefore, becomes exposed to the oral environment. The exposed cementum may be lost or it may be influenced by environmental factors. These conditions are not discussed here, because they are not considered to be age changes per second however, the clinical implications of such changes must not be overlooked in geriatric dentistry.

The most characteristic age change in cementum is the gradual increase in thickness. Cementum deposition occurs throughout life. The total width of the cementum almost triples between the ages of 10 and 75 years. Hypercementosis may affect one or more teeth. It is a pathological condition that may be caused by local factors. Certain systemic conditions may also be characterized by hypercementosis, such as Paget's disease. These features are important in the differential diagnosis of increased cementum formation.

Dentin

Two age-dependent changes take place in dentin: continued growth, referred to as physiological secondary dentin formation and gradual obturation of the dentinal tubules, referred to as dentin sclerosis. These processes occur concomitantly, but they are independent.

Physiological or regular secondary dentin formation is a continuation of the dentinogenesis after the tooth is fully formed. The same odontoblasts that formed the primary dentin are considered to continue matrix formation at a slow rate. The odontoblasts in old teeth are fewer and shorter than in young teeth. No distinct demarcation is found between primary dentin and physiological secondary dentin using ordinary histological techniques, but the structure gradually becomes more irregular, probably due to the crowding of the odontoblasts. The number of dentinal tubules is reduced, and their course is somewhat more irregular than in primary dentin. The predentin width increases with age, possibly due to a slow rate of mineralization of secondary dentin. However, special techniques may differentiate quite clearly between the primary land secondary dentin, for example, by evaluating the distribution of organic material in demineralized sections. The formation of secondary dentin reduces the pulp chamber. This reduction in size does not affect the pulp chamber evenly, and it varies for different types of teeth. For molars, relatively more dentin forms on the ceiling and floor of the pulp chamber than on the side walls. On upper incisors, more secondary dentin forms on the palatal side of the pulp chamber than elsewhere. In impacted teeth, secondary dentin formation apparently stars in the apical region and proceeds coronally.

Obturation of the tubules by gradual growth of the peritubular dentin is a typical age change. It results in a change in the refractive index of the dentin, making it more translucent, hence the term transparent dentin. Weber indicates that only about half the tubules become completely obturated under physiological mineralized peritubular dentin or obturated tubules in the most pulpal part of the primary dentin or in the secondary dentin must be regarded as age changes, because they are not present as primary structures; that is, these portions of the dentin form without the presence of highly mineralized peritubular dentin.

The age changes in dentin are important clinically. The obturation of the tubules leads to a reduction in the sensitivity of the tissue. Furthermore, the adhesive properties of aged, cervical dentin are different from those of young dentin, which is important to keep in mind when restoring Class V lesions on old individuals. A reduction in the dentin permeability is also important to prevent the ingress of toxic agents. The addition of more bulk to the dentin may be important to prevent pulp reactions and even pulp exposure, especially which associated with heavy attrition, in which a considerable portion of the dentin is lost.

Pulp

The dental pulp in teeth from old individuals differs from that in younger teeth by having more fibers and fewer cells. It is difficult to ascertain how many of these changes are age-dependent per se and which are caused by the function of the teeth or pathological processes. Atrophy of the pulp tissue described in old literature dealing with structure of the dental pulp was probably not caused by age changes but by histological artifacts.

The blood supply apparently decreases with age; at least, the number of arteries entering the apical foramen does. Studies indicated that the number of branches of blood vessels was markedly reduced with age, including the branching in the subodontoblastic region. These changes are clinically important because the pulp in older individuals cannot be expected to have the same reparative capacities as that in young teeth. Thus, pulp-capping procedures or pulpotomies must be expected to have a lower success rate in old individuals; that is, repair by dentin bridge formation should not be expected. The cross-linking between collagen fibers in the pulp decreases with age, and the calcium content increase.

Electron microscopy of old pulps in cats has shown loss and degeneration of both myelinated and unmyelinated nerves compared with pulps in young individuals. A marked decrease in pulpal calcitonin-gene related peptide and substance P-like immunore-

activity was also demonstrated. These findings may explain the reduced sensitivity in teeth from older individuals. It is also likely that these age changes noted in the nerves affect the healing capacity of the pulp in old individuals.

The presence of pulp stones has been attributed to pathological changes, but they have also been considered as age changes. Hall maintained that 6%–7% of normal pulps exhibit mineralization of various types, while about 75% of the pulps from teeth with pathological lesions (mainly caries or deep restorations) showed such changes. A 1:10 ratio of pulpal mineralization in noncarious teeth has been reported in young and old individuals. It appears likely, therefore, that pathological processes are more important for pulp stone formation than age. The type of mineralization may be important in this context; thus, studies indicated that denticle formation does not increase with age, but diffuse mineralization does increase in frequency. This observation has later been confirmed.

Conclusion

Limited information is available on age changes in teeth. Macroscopic changes include alteration in form due to wear and attrition and in color due to secondary dentin formation, pigmentation and altered patterns of light reflection.

The surface enamel exhibits certain acquired properties, such as the increase in fluoride content, which builds up slowly with age. The number of enamel cracks or acquired lamellae also increases with age.

The cementum increases in thickness with age, which results in a degeneration of the cementocytes in the deep layers of the tissue. Furthermore, the number of repaired resorption defects and the fluoride and magnesium content increase. Gingival recession leads to the exposure of the cementum to the oral environment.

Age changes in dentin constitute two independent processes, secondary dentin formation and obturation of dentinal tubules. The main pulp changes include a change from a cell-rich connective tissue. The pulp blood supply is reduced with age and diffuse mineralization increase.

11. 1. 2 Age Changes in the Oral Mucous Membranes and Periodontium

Although some clinical changes have been reported in the appearance of the oral mucosa with age, little is known about changes in its functional capacities with age. In addition, most reports of age-associated mucosal changes have not carefully controlled for secondary factors such as general health. The results of studies of age-associated changes in the structure and cell kinetics of the epithelial and connective tissue components of the mucosa have failed to produce a clear picture of underlying cellular changes. In the connective tissue of the gingival, palatal mucosa and periodontal ligament, the ability of the fibroblasts to synthesize new collagen decreases with age. Under the light microscope, the collagen fibers appear thicker and coarser, giving the tissue a fibrotic appearance, but studies of the concentration of collagen have produced conflicting results and inconclusive findings. The rate of conversion of soluble collagen to insoluble collagen increases with age and, correspondingly, the denaturing temperature is higher for collagen in the gingival of old than of young individuals. These changes may affect the functional properties of the periodontal tissues in the aged. However, there are no reasons to suggest that age-related alterations in the periodontium may be manifested as loss of probing attachment or alveolar bone.

11.1.3 Changes in Salivary Glands and Salivary Secretion with Aging

Many recent studies have indicated that there is no generalized diminution in salivary gland performance with increased age. It would appear that previous suggestions of age-related changes primarily reflected disease- or therapy-induced alterations. Since saliva is critically important to the maintenance of oral health, any general disturbance in salivary gland function would result in severe morbidity. Clinicians must take care not to ascribe casually to aging the complaints by older patients that suggest salivary gland disorders but rather to consider age as a possible contributory factor increasing patient vulnerability.

11.2 Medical and Pharmacological Issues in the Dental Care of Older Adults

11.2.1 Medical Issues in the Dental Care of Older Adults

In terms of overall health and functional status, the older adult population is quite heterogeneous, ranging from those who are free of significant disease and disability to those with complex health problems, physical impairments, and medication regimens. However, as patients live longer with significant chronic disease, and as older patient seek dental care, practitioners will more likely encounter medically and functionally compromised individuals. And while dentistry is commonly viewed as a primary care discipline, since patients usually present without referral from another health care provider, modern dental practice is also a technically sophisticated, procedure-oriented discipline centered on restoring and maintaining the health of a specific region of the body. Because of this focus and the array of conditions that older individuals seeking dental care may manifest, effective communication between dental providers and primary physicians is crucial to ensure that dental treatment provided to the compromised elderly is safe.

Indications for medical consultation

Dentals should not view physician consultation in terms of seeking permission to render indicated dental care. It is assumed that the dentist is practicing within his or her realm of professional expertise. Furthermore, physicians receive little training in dental therapeutics and are unlikely to know how a dentist plans and delivers specific treatments such as dental extractions, endodontic therapy, or operative dental procedures.

Dentists should consider consulting with physicians for three basic reasons. First, dentists may have questions about the accuracy of the medical history or medication regimen provided by a patient. Second, dentistry may have specific concerns regarding the ability of a patient to tolerate a proposed course of treatment. Finally, dentists can provide physicians with significant information regarding the potential relationship between oral health problems or interventions and systemic health.

11.2.2 Pharmacology and Aging

Our understanding of disease processes continues to progress, leading to the development of more effective and potent drug modalities. It is no surprise that older adults, who have the highest prevalence of chronic diseases, are the principal consumers of these potent drugs. Drug use in the elderly is two-edged sword; it can provide a cure or a palliative treatment of disease in a safe and cost-effective manner, or can be a major source of morbidity, and even mortality. This paradox is accentuated in elderly people due to age-related changes in physiological status, as well as multiple diseases with associated polypharmacy. Therefore, it is important to realize both the advantages and limitations of the drugs prescribed to older patients.

In every case the dentist must carefully review the patient's medical history, including medication usage, and consider the potential benefit versus the potential risk of each prescribed drug. This section focuses primarily on the pharmacokinetic aspects of the medications prescribed by dentists that are particularly relevant and important for the care of elderly patients in the dental office. Although it is also pertinent to consider potential pharmacodynamic changes that emerge in older individuals, as discussed previously, current studies have been able to characterize only a restricted number of pharmacodynamic shifts in elderly people. While a few investigations have identified changes in the pharmacodynamic response of a limited number of agents, the ability to distinguish the physiological changes induced by drugs in the elderly is significantly complicated by the interplay of age-related diminished functional reserve, multiple disease states, polypharmacy, dietary factors, and compliance. Despite the paucity of pharmacodynamic information, changes in the mechanism of drug action in the elderly are reported when data are available. In summary, this section provides a broad overview of the pharmacokinetic properties of common pharmacological drug classes typically prescribed by the dental practitioner.

11.3　Dental Caries and Pulp Diseases in the Aging Individual

11.3.1　Root Surface Caries

With increasing age, gingival recedes gradually and root surfaces become exposed to the oral environment in most individuals. The distribution of gingival recession within the dentition among 60-year-old and 70-year-old is demonstrated. In principle, recession occurs on all surfaces and is not associated with mechanical tooth cleaning only, although it is most pronounced on buccal surfaces(Color Figure 11-1).

The root surface may be more vulnerable to mechanical destruction than the enamel because the structure and chemical composition of cementum and dentin differ. Thus, in populations with a tradition for regular oral hygiene procedures, the cementum layer is frequently abraded away, exposing the dentin. This phenomenon is particularly pronounced

when root surfaces are regularly care professionals. Therefore, the clinical term root caries may cover caries lesions in the cementum but lesions occur mostly in the root dentin.

Diagnosing, preventing and choosing appropriate treatment for root surface caries requires basic knowledge of the clinical appearance, epidemiological features, histopathology and microbiology of the disease. These aspects are therefore discussed in detail in the following sections.

Clinical features of root surface caries

Root surface caries comprises a continuum of changes ranging from needle-point small, slightly softened and discolored spots on the root to extensive, brownish or very dark soft areas encircling the entire toot surface. Sometimes cavities even extend into the pulp chamber.

This section describes the most typical appearance of what are designated active and inactive root surface caries lesions, and some diagnostic criteria to be used both in epidemiological studies and in daily clinical praxis are suggested.

Unlike the initial enamel lesion, the early stages of root surface caries appear as one of more small well-defined discolored areas, predominantly located at the cemento-enamel junction. The active lesions are yellowish of light brown in color and frequently covered by a microbial deposit that may wary considerably in thickness. The carious tissue feels soft on slight probing. In slowly progressing lesions the surface may be brownish to black, and the consistency feels leathery. These changes may occur without obvious cavitation. When cavitation occurs, the margins are frequently sharp and irregular.

The lesions tend to spread laterally and often coalesce with minor neighboring lesions. The lesions may eventually encircle the tooth, in particular when they are located along the cemento-enamel junction. It is of interest that the lesions rarely seen to extend in an apical direction as the gingival margin recedes. New lesions develop instead at the level of the gingival margin. This may occur irrespective of an inactive lesion being located more coronally.

The inactive lesion is typically dark brown, often almost black. The surface is frequently shiny, smooth and hard on probing. This applies whether the lesion exhibits a frank cavity with distinct loss of tissue or not. However, if cavitation has occurred the margins most often appear smooth. In case of longstanding inactive lesions, the root surface may appear glossy and only discoloration suggests previous caries activity.

In addition to these common types of lesions predominating in individuals who perform regular oral hygiene and frequently visit a dentist, case may occur in which almost the entire exposed root surface is covered by a clinically distinct layer of plaque; after removal, this reveals an underlying darkly discolored leathery root surface, virtually without macroscopic signs of cavitation. These types of lesions have been observed in elderly patients exhibiting impaired salivary secretion as a result of medication or in patients who are unable to perform proper oral hygiene for various reasons.

This distinction between inactive and active root surface lesions is of clinical importance, as it shows that root surfaces react to the dynamic processes taking place at the plaque-root surface interface due to intermittent pH changes. If these processes are interfered with by, for instance, regular plaque removal, active lesions may become arrested and converted to inactive lesions. Such a distinction is useful in recording the oral health status of the individual, as it gives an immediate measure of previous caries challenges as well as an indication of the need for active professional intervention at the time of examination.

11.3.2 *Pathology and Treatment of Disease of the Pulp*

Traditionally, teeth in older individuals have been considered "a good risk" for operative procedures. Today it is generally accepted that age reduce the functional capacity of a tissue. Nevertheless, there seems to be agreement that teeth in mature individuals react to restorative procedures in the same way as young teeth. The prognosis of endodontic treatment is not influenced by the age of the patient. The exception may be pulp-capping, as there is some evidence that age may affect the outcome of the treatment unfavorably.

Although there has been a growing literature on the prevalence of root caries in older patients, the impact of root caries on the need for—and complications associated with-endodontic treatment in the elderly has not been researched adequately.

Thus, in pulpal pathosis, the same guidelines should apply for planning of dental care in older as in younger people:

    Adequate nutrition.
    Good oral hygiene.

    Fluorides.
    Necessary dental treatment.

Prevention is also the key word in this group of patients. If the patients have difficulty maintaining adequate or hygiene, professional cleaning at frequent intervals is an effective way to prevent disease. Fluoride-containing toothpaste is a must and can often with advantage be supplemented by local application of fluorides, especially in patients who tend to develop root caries. Restorative dentistry should be performed with normal biological considerations. A base should be used in cavities of old teeth as well as in young teeth. Marginal leakage can be largely prevented by the use of a varnish under amalgam restoration and by using the acid-etch technique when resin fillings are inserted. Technique when resin fillings are inserted. Pulp-capping or pulpotomy procedures are generally contraindicated in older patients. Teeth with pulp exposure should be treated with pulpectomy and root canal filling. As already mentioned, the prognosis of this treatment is excellent, as is the prognosis of root canal treatment of teeth with necrotic pulps in older patients.

Conclusion

Over the years, external infectious, toxic or iatrogenic irritants cause irreversible changes in the endodontium. Certain systemic factors may have an effect as well. The changes include intratubular dentin formation of dentinal sclerosis, secondary dentin and intrapulpal hard tissue formation, a reduction in the number of cells, capillaries and nerves, and an increase in the quantity of collagen fibers. However, the pulp may maintain its identity throughout life and remain in a functional state if necessary dental treatment is rendered.

The same guidelines apply for dental treatment of pulpal pathosis in older as in younger patients. Prevention of disease, especially the maintenance of good oral hygiene, is the key to good oral health in elderly people as in all other population groups.

11.4 Aging and Periodontal Disease

Prevalence and severity

Periodontal diseases are among the most prevalent chronic conditions in dentate older populations. Several epidemiological surveys have found that the prevalence and severity of periodontal diseases increase with age. One of these studies found that periodontal attachment loss increased progressively with age, whereas the proportion of individuals with gingival bleeding remained relatively constant for each decade of adult life. Only a week correlation between pocket depth and ascending age was observed. Comparable data have been reported in other studies. One of these described the prevalence of periodontal diseased in a well-defined, selected, population of 22- to 90-year-old healthy individuals who were nonsmokers and not taking prescription medications. The results revealed higher percentages of tooth surfaces with dental plaque, gingival bleeding, calculus, recession and attachment loss in the oldest age group as compared with the young and middle-aged groups. Mean periodontal pocket depths increased slightly with age, but only the youngest and the oldest age groups differed significantly.

In summary, the evidence indicates that elderly people living in nursing homes have more severe periodontal conditions and poorer elderly people. This trend has been explained by the higher degree of helplessness among nursing home residents. In addition, oral health often assumes a lower priority among the frail elderly than does other aspects of their physical health. Other barriers may be the mobility status of the patient, the availability of dental services and the accessibility of the dental office. Financial constraints may also play a role. Furthermore, systemic diseases, medications and such conditions as drug-in-hygiene and make the tissue more vulnerable to periodontal diseases.

Susceptibility to periodontal disease

Enhanced severity of periodontal diseases with age has been related to the length of time the periodontal tissues have been exposed to the dentogingival bacterial plaque and is considered to reflect the individual's cumulative oral history (Color Figure 11-2). However, the susceptibility of the periodontium to plaque-induced periodontal breakdown may be influenced by the aging process of buy the specific health problems of the aging patient. Knowledge of the tissue changes that occur during aging is therefore not only essential for understanding the basic pathophysiological features of aging but is also of great clinical significance in planning treatment and in evaluating the prognosis of the treatment chosen for the elderly patient,

Aging reduces the ability of the individual to adapt to environmental stress. At the biological level, aging is associated with changes that lead to a progressive, irreversible deterioration of the func-

tional capacities of several tissues and organs. Changes in structure and function during aging may affect the host response to plaque microorganisms and may influence the rate of periodontal destruction in older people. Although age changes in the periodontal tissues have been investigated extensively, there is less information on the response of the periodontium of older humans to microbial infection.

The studies concerned with determining the influence of aging the development of gingival inflammation have produced conflicting results. Nevertheless, most of the investigations reviewed have shown that the host response to plaque microorganisms changes with increasing age, manifested by a more pronounced inflammatory reaction in the gingival. On the other hand, the age factor may be overruled by the susceptibility to periodontal breakdown. It has not been shown, however, that the rate of progression of periodontitis involving the deeper parts of the periodontium is different in young and old subjects. On the contrary, periodontitis is usually considered to progress slowly in elderly subjects. The increased intensity of the inflammatory reaction in the gingival of older people may therefore reflect a local defense mechanism by which the host attempts to compensate for a less effective immune response or, perhaps, for a decline in the effectiveness of polymorphonuclear leukocytes and monocytes in phagocytosis.

Prognosis

Prognosis is a prediction of the probable course or a disease and of the prospect for prospect for recovery. It includes evaluation of the natural history of the disease without treatment as well as assessment of the anticipated response to treatment.

The prognosis for periodontal therapy is generally considered to be better for elderly than for younger individuals if an equal amount of periodontal attachment loss has occurred, because periodontal destruction has progressed at a much slower rate in the older person. Therefore, the past history, that is, the duration of the disease, or the length of time during which the periodontal tissues have been exposed to the dentogingival plaque, may be important in estimating the prognosis. In principle, a moderate attachment loss in a young subject can be regarded as a rather serious situation, whereas a corresponding degree of periodontal destruction in an elderly patient can be considered less serious.

Despite these general guidelines, it should not be overlooked that periodontal diseases are often very selective. Substantial destruction may occur in some teeth and little or none in others. The overall prognosis of the dentition depends on, but may differ from that of individual teeth.

The altered host response and the reduced healing capacity in elderly subjects can be compensated for by reducing the bacterial impact. The ability of the elderly patient to heal so well suggests that the healing capacity is far in excess of what is needed for normal tissue healing. Adequate plaque control is of paramount importance and can be achieved. However, in patients who are not proficient in oral hygiene, the altered biological responses may imply an increased risk for complications and progression of periodontitis.

Periodontal treatment and prophylaxis

In periodontal care for elderly people, the usual practice has been to postpone treatment and adopt a holding pattern until the patient was considered ready for complete dentures. Old patients were looked at with reluctance by many dentists, and periodontal treatment and more complex restorations were often not considered. This attitude to treat of older people was based on the idea that the elderly patient could not endure periodontal treatment which included surgery, that the prognosis for the treatment was poor or simply that complex therapy was unwarranted since the person had only a few years left to live. It was not based on the range of the therapeutic options afforded to other patients.

Older people are increasingly likely to have chronic impairments or even more serious disabilities or diseases that may adversely affect periodontal health. Frail and functionally dependent elderly people constitute a high-risk population base on complex health problems and functional status, which may seriously influence oral health and related treatment. This group also includes patients who are unable to carry out adequate oral hygiene, and anyone on daily medication that produces xerostomia as a side effect. Therefore, these subgroups of elderly need to be especially targeted for prevention.

Approaches to treatment

The aim of periodontal treatment is to eliminate or control gingivitis and to arrest the progression of periodontitis by removing the microbial plaque.

Conservative therapy consisting of frequent tooth cleaning and repeated individualized instruction in oral hygiene techniques constitutes an appropriate therapeutic approach. In cases in which the clinician

considers it unlikely that complete removal of soft and hard bacterial deposits from infected root surfaces will be achieved by scaling and root planning alone, periodontal surgery may be necessary to create access for proper debridement. A second indication for periodontal surgery is to establish a gingival morphology that facilitates the patient's self-performed postoperative plaque control.

The age of the patient is no contraindication to periodontal surgery. For instance, a robust 80-year-old may be an excellent candidate for maximum treatment. On the other hand, the outcome in terms of tooth longevity may not outweigh the trauma of surgical treatment to a frail elderly patient.

Complicated surgical management requires knowledge of and deference to the general health status of the patient, the altered tissue responses and healing. The principles for periodontal surgery are basically the same for adults of any age, and there are no real differences between the surgical procedures used in young and old people. To minimize patient discomfort and reduce the risk of postoperative complications, surgery should be performed as atraumatically as possible. Available evidence clearly demonstrates that excellent wound healing can be obtained in elderly people. Provided of the tissues are handled properly.

Consultation with the elderly patient's physician is often necessary prior to treatment to clarify specific aspects of his or her medical problems and/or medications. Patients with valvular heart disease should receive antibiotic chemoprophylaxis prior to scaling and surgery to prevent infection by hematogenous spread.

In medically and/or mentally compromised elderly patients, nonsurgical periodontal therapy may be the best approach to treatment. In old individuals who are in poor health, the aims of treatment should be to keep the patient free of pain and infection and to maintain the dentition in a functional condition for life. Subjective oral well-being should be the leading concept in treatment planning. A primary goal must be that the trauma of does not exceed the gains of treatment. Therefore, in individual cases the clinician may have to modify the treatment plan to include procedures appropriate for the specific patient.

Conclusion

The rates of edentulism and tooth loss are rapidly declining. Therefore, the numbers of old individuals requiring periodontal treatment will most likely increase. Prevention and treatment of periodontal disease in elderly subjects require dental services based on improved knowledge of the biology and pathology of the periodontium. Periodontal care for elderly people involves a complete analysis of the physical and emotional status of the patient. Age changes may affect the assessment of the periodontal problem, the treatment plan, its prognosis and the risk for complications following therapy. Available evidence clearly demonstrates that periodontal diseases can be treated successfully in the elderly and that periodontal health can be sustained.

11.5 Oral and Maxillofacial Surgery for the Geriatric Patient

The scope of oral and maxillofacial surgery for the elderly patient is similar to that for the younger adult in terms of the specific procedures that may be indicated. Nevertheless, the presence of systemic disease and nutritional deficiency, the use of multiple pharmaceutical preparations, and other sequelae of aging make each elderly surgery patient a unique case, with special needs in terms of medical management as well as surgery.

Medical evaluation

As with all patients, the surgical treatment of the elderly patient begins with medical history. A survey of over 4000 patients showed that approximately 65% of patients over age 60 years had multiple positive responses to a health history questionnaire, as compared with 16% multiple positive response in patients under 30 years, likewise, 40% of those over 60 years were taking more than one type of medication, as compared with only 6% of those under 30 years. Consequently, although thorough evaluation of the medical history is essential prior to initiating surgery for any patient, particular attention must be paid to the health status of the elderly individual.

Obtaining accurate health history information cannot be relegated to the review of a written questionnaire. Although most dentists use self-administered questionnaires, responses to written questions have been shown to be notoriously inaccurate, as illustrated by one study of over 2000 health histories in which one-third of all patients, regardless of age or of individual health status, gave inaccurate answers. In the same study, 11% of 675 patients who were in poor health replied "yes" to the question, "Are you in good health?" Thus, although a questionnaire may be useful, it must be supplemented by a follow-up dialogue history by the dentist. For

some patients, confirmation of physical status with the patient's physician is also indicated.

This questionnaire is applicable to all patients, regardless of age. For elderly patients, particular attention should be given to the cardiovascular and pulmonary systems, since the incidence of cardiopulmonary compromise increase with age. Detailed questioning regarding medications is also necessary since some elderly patients, on various drugs for years, may not view them as important and fail to mention them on a written questionnaire. For patients intended to undergo surgery, specific questioning regarding intake of aspirin the clotting mechanism is indicated. Likewise, for this group, an evaluation of nutritional intake is also important, since the incidence of infection and of poor healing is greater in the nutritionally compromised patient. Acquired disorders of the immune system are currently less common in this age group, but general questions regarding the immune system are acceptable in all age groups.

Surgical procedures

The majority of oral surgical procedures for the geriatric patient fall into the categories of extractions and preprosthetic surgery. Complete radiographic surveys including panoramic view are recommended to rule out occult pathological conditions. In this age group, impacted teeth should be removed only if concomitant pathological conditions are present. Isolated maxillary molar teeth are often in close approximation to the sinus, and consideration should be given to surgical sectioning to avoid the complication of oroantral fistula.

Conclusion

Surgery for the geriatric patient encompasses the entire spectrum of oral and maxillofacial surgery. Consideration of medical conditions, medications, and the altered physiology of the aged, as well as individualization of treatment modalities form the cornerstones of care for this patient population.

11.6 Prosthetic Considerations in Geriatric Dentistry

Oral status and treatment needs

Oral health and oral care are important to maintain proper mastication, digestion, speech, appearance and psychological wellbeing. The pattern of use of dental services and the need and demand for dental treatment are clearly different in elderly and younger populations. Thus, in many industrialized societies more than 50% of the elderly population is edentulous. Furthermore, there seems to be a significant discrepancy between the objective need and the demand for prosthetic and dental and dental care. Thus, many elderly people do not visit dentists regularly, and those with the lowest income and the least education are two or three times less likely to see a dentist than those with the most education and the highest income. Nevertheless, future elderly populations are expected to become increasingly aware of the important of a well-functioning masticatory system. Thus, although the number of complete or partially edentulous people is decreasing, this may not necessarily reduce the demand for prosthetic treatment and services.

Future prosthetic treatments may be more differentiated and perhaps also more complicated. The presence of some natural teeth tends to favor treatment plans that preserve these teeth, as they are important tor the retention and stabilization of a removable denture. Great care should also be taken to design removable dentures with the fewest harmful effects and to see patients regularly to check the functioning of the masticatory system and oral hygiene. The fact that people tend to postpone the acquisition of removable dentures until late in life may account for marked difficulties could be partly overcome by installing implant-retained fixed bridges or removable complete dentures. However, chronic debilitating physical, medical or emotional problems may completely jeopardize the prognosis of such treatments if regular oral health care is not available.

Diagnosis and treatment planning

A careful history and clinical examination of the elderly person are essential in attempting to clarify this person's demand and need for prosthetic treatment. Also, it is important to consider systemic and local factors as well as the person's previous experience with dentures before deciding on treatment and establishing prognosis.

Conclusion

The outcome of prosthetic treatment in geriatric dentistry is determined by several factors such as the general and oral health status of the patient, the patient's degree of cooperation, the financial resources available for care, the biological and technical quality of prosthetic materials and the prosthodontist's knowledge, judgment and technical ability. Thus, insight into the clinical and technical aspects of prosthetic treatment is important to be able to successfully treat elderly people who are partially or totally edentulous. However, the greatest challenge to the clinician is to choose between treating the patient, with the risk of producing iatrogenic disease, and not treating the patient, with the risk of more damage occurring to the masticatory system.

▪ Summary

A vast number of scientific articles on the psychosocial and somatic needs of the aging microorganism, and their clinical implications, have been published in more and more journal.

It is now time for summation and interpretation.

Thus, important objectives of this chapter are to provide to the reader a comprehensive and convenient account of the complex issues of aging, to produce and assembly of the current concepts of systemic and oral disorders in the aging patient, and present the means to their solution or amelioration, with the full realization that these challenges can only be met by basic knowledge and clinical competence.

It has been said that the evolution of a profession is evidenced by the scope and quality of its literature. It is our hope that this text might be a small contribution to this principle. However, the merit of this chapter lies in the wide expanse and penetration depth.

▪ Questions

1. What changes are there in the tooth with aging?

2. What medical issues do the elderly have in the dental care of older adult?

3. What characteristics are root surface caries in the aging individual?

4. What susceptibilities to periodontal disease are there in older adults?

5. How important will medical evaluation have in oral and maxillofacial surgery for the geriatric patient?

6. How diagnoses and treatment planning will you considerate in geriatric dentistry for the elderly prosthetic?

(Zhaochen Shan　单兆臣)

References

[1] Bhussry BR, Hess WC. Aging of enamel and dentin. J Gerontol, 1963, 18(4): 343-344.

[2] Arends J, Jongebloed WL, Schuthof J. Crystallite diameters of enamel near the anatomical surface. An investigation of mature, deciduous and monerupted human enamel. Caries Res, 1983, 17(2): 97-110.

[3] Henry JI, Weinmann MD. The pattern of resorption and repair of human cementum. J Assoc, 1951, 42(3): 270-290.

[4] Nakata TM, Stepnick RJ, Zipkin I. Chemistry of human dental cementum: the effect of age and fluoride exposure on the concentrations of ash, fluoride, calcium, phosphorus and magnesium. J Periodontol, 1972, 43(2): 115-124.

[5] Nitzan DW, Michaeli Y, Weireb M, et al. The effect on aging on tooth morphology: a study of impacted teeth. Oral Surg Oral Med Oral Pathol, 1986, 61(1): 54-60.

[6] Mjor IA. Relationship between microradiography and stainability of human coronal dentine. Arch Oral Biol, 1966, 11(12): 1317-1323.

[7] Nielsen CJ, Bentley JP, Marshall FJ. Age changes of the vascular pattern of the human dental collagen. Arch Oral Biol, 1983, 28(8): 759-764.

[8] Sterrett JD, Lindhe J, Berghlund T. Epithelial remnants in the crestal periodontium of the dog. J Clin Periodontol, 1993, 19(2): 138-142.

[9] Levy AM, Jakobsen JR. A comparison of medical histories reported by dental patients and their physicians, Spec Care Dent, 1991, 11(1): 26-31.

[10] Ouslander JG. Drug therapy in the elderly. Ann intern med, 1981, 95(6): 711-722.

[11] Abernethy DR. Methodological concerns for clinical trials in geriatrics: benzodazepines. In: Culture NR, Narang PK. Drugs studies in the elderly: methodological concerns. New York: Plenum Book Co. , 1986: 189-205.

[12] Nyvad B, Fejerskov O. Active root surface caries converted into in active caries as a response to oral hygiene. Scand J Dent Res, 1986, 94(3): 281-284.

[13] Disney JA, Stamm JW, Graves RC, et al. Description and preliminary results of a caries risk assessment model. University of North Carolina Dental Ecology, 1990: 215-217.

[14] Westbrook JL, Miller AS, Chilton NW, et al. Root surface caries: a clinical, histopathologic and microradiographic investigation. Caries Res, 1974, 8(3): 249-255.

[15] Saotome Y, Tada A, Hanada N, et al. Relationship of cariogenic bacteria levels with periodontal status and root surface caries in elderly Japanese. Gerodontology, 2006, 23(4): 219-225.

[16] Ship JA, Wolf A. Gingival and periodontal parameters in a population of healthy adults, 22 - 90 years of age. Gerodotology, 1988, 7(2): 55-60.

[17] Pedrazzoli V, Killian M, Karring T, et al. Effect of surgical and non-surgical periodontal treatment of periodontal status and subgingival microbiota. J Clin Periodontol, 1991, 18(8): 598-604.

[18] Paranhos HF, Silva CH, Venezian GC, et al. Distribution of biofilm on internal and external surfaces of upper complete dentures: the effect of hygiene instruction. Gerodontology, 2007, 24(3): 162-168.

[19] Freedman KA. Management of the geriatric dental patient. Chicago: Quintessence Publishing, 1979: 87-96.

[20] Baxter JC. Nutrition and the geriatric edentulous patient. Spec Care Dent, 1981, 1(6): 259-261.

Chapter

12

Oral Manifestations of Systemic Diseases

▪ Objectives

The objective of the chapter is to provide a general overview of conditions that have oral manifestations but also involve other organ systems. Its target audiences are undergraduate and postgraduate students as well as practicing clinicians.

▪ Key Concepts

There are hundreds of lesions or diseases that occur primarily within the oral cavity. Lesions in the mouth are also associated with a variety of systemic diseases. These lesions may be useful adjuncts to the clinical diagnosis of a syndrome and occasionally can be the presenting sign or symptom of a systemic disease. This chapter discusses the more common oral lesions associated with extraoral disease.

▪ Introduction

The oral cavity is an important anatomical location with a role in many critical physiologic processes, such as digestion, respiration, and speech. It is also unique for the presence of exposed hard tissue surrounded by mucosa. Most systemic diseases can affect the oral cavity. Some oral changes are nonspecific, whereas others directly lead to the diagnosis of a particular disorder. A systems approach is used here to catalog these oral changes.

This article is not intended to provide details about the diagnosis and management of all of these conditions in detail. All conditions described in this article have excellent full-length medicine entries, many of which are linked herein, that should be consulted for comprehensive information.

12. 1   HIV Disease

In the 20 years since the onset of the HIV pandemic, a number of oral and cutaneous entities have been recognized to be associated with HIV disease. Importantly, note that no unique condition specific to HIV disease has been identified in the oral cavity. These conditions have all been described in patients with other forms of immunocompromise and, indeed, in immunocompetent individuals. However, the clinical presentation is often more severe or atypical in patients with HIV disease. Many patients have both oral and cutaneous conditions simultaneously. Most of these conditions seldom manifest with CD4 counts lower than 400 cells/μL, and many have a positive predictive value for immune decline.

The most frequent oral lesions were hairy leukoplakia (18.7%), thrush (6.6%) or erythematous candidosis (2.1%), Kaposi's sarcoma (1.6%) and oral ulcers (2%). Overall, the tongue is the reported site of oral manifestations and it has been found to be involved in 75% of patients dying from AIDS. Tongue lesions include any of those described below, but there may also be nonspecific glossitis or melanotic pigmentation. However, the frequency of such lesions varies in other groups. Kaposi's sarcoma and hairy leukoplakia, for example, are disproportionately frequent in men who have sex with men. The most common of these entities are discussed below.

12. 1. 1   Candidiasis

Oral candidiasis is often the first presenting sign of HIV infection. HIV infection should be considered in patients presenting with repeated oral candidiasis in the absence of other associated risk factors, such as steroid or antibiotic use.

The 4 common classifications of candidal infections are ① pseudomembranous candidiasis, ② erythematous candidiasis, ③ angular cheilitis, and ④ hyperplastic candidiasis. Pseudomembranous candidiasis is the most common presentation in HIV-infected individuals. This is characterized by white or whitish-yellow papules that can be wiped from the oral mucosa to reveal erosions or erythematous mucosa. These often manifest on the buccal mucosa, palate, and vestibule, although any surface may be involved.

Erythematous candidiasis is more difficult to diagnose because it manifests as a nonspecific area of erythema, commonly on the palate or dorsum of the tongue (or both as a result of autoinoculation). Hyperplastic candidiasis is uncommon and manifests as adherent white plaques that cannot be easily removed. These are often mistaken for premalignant

leukoplakia. Angular cheilitis appears as cracked, red, and sometimes ulcerated fissures in the corners of the mouth with or without intraoral symptoms. Although the history and physical examination findings help establish the diagnosis, confirmation can be made by using a potassium hydroxide (KOH) preparation, which shows hyphae, pseudohyphae, or spores. The KOH preparation is often negative in persons with erythematous candidiasis or angular cheilitis. If confirmation is required, cytology or tissue biopsy can also be used, with the latter test being definitive.

The frequency of candidal infection increases as HIV disease progresses (i. e. as viral loads increase and CD4 lymphocyte counts decline). Antifungal treatment is often effective, but the condition can be difficult to eradicate in immunocompromised patients. Often, this is because clinical recovery does not coincide with mycologic recovery; the patient may appear well but still may be harboring fungal organisms. Additionally, fungal resistance to azole drugs (e. g. fluconazole) is increased among HIV-infected patients. If patients do not respond, culture and sensitivity studies should be considered. Finally, patients must also remember to treat any removable dental prosthesis, such as dentures, because these can act as fomites and can reinoculate the patient.

12. 1. 2   Hairy Leukoplakia

Hairy leukoplakia (HL) manifests as corrugated white plaques most commonly on the lateral portions of the tongue. These plaques can range in appearance from very thin and homogenous to a thickened, rough area that mimics hyperplastic candidiasis. The infectious agent responsible for these lesions is Epstein-Barr virus (EBV), located within the epithelial cells. In the early 1980s, HL was first identified and characterized in patients who were HIV positive, but it has also been described in persons with other states of immunocompromise (e. g. renal transplant recipients).

HL remains the most specific manifestation of HIV disease to occur in the mouth, and its presence has prognostic implications for the progression to AIDS because patients rarely manifest the condition with CD4 counts greater than 200 μL. The white verrucous plaques vary greatly in size, are not premalignant, and are usually asymptomatic. These lesions can be clinically mistaken for candidiasis, and a biopsy should be performed for definitive diagnosis.

Histologically, hairlike folds can be seen, which demonstrate hyperparakeratosis, acanthosis, and groups of ballooning cells, with little inflammatory infiltrate present. Definitive diagnosis may be made with in situ hybridization of the DNA from EBV in surface epithelial cells.

Although the severity of HL is not directly correlated with HIV stage, HL has been shown to precede the diagnosis of AIDS in patients with HIV infection, and it appears to be a prognostic indicator of advanced disease and death within several years. An analysis of 198 patients with HL in the pre-highly active antiretroviral therapy (HAART) demonstrated that the median time to onset of AIDS was 24 months and to death was 41 months. Oral HL may be the presenting sign in as many as 5% of patients who are HIV positive. Because HL is usually asymptomatic, treatment is elective. HL responds to antiviral medication, such as oral acyclovir, but lesions generally recur after cessation of therapy. If a patient reports symptoms associated with HL, the lesions are most likely superinfected with Candida species. Antifungal treatment usually ameliorates the symptoms.

12. 1. 3 Kaposi's Sarcoma

Among patients with AIDS, Kaposi's sarcoma (KS) is mainly seen in men who have sex with men and, in some areas of the USA, for example, it has become the most common malignant tumor of the oral cavity. It is also very occasionally seen in HIV-negative immunosuppressed organ transplant patients. AIDS-type KS is associated with a high rate of second neoplasms, particularly lymphomas and clinical suspicion of the diagnosis of KS is also strengthened by coexisting or a history of opportunistic infections.

KS is a neoplasm that was extremely uncommon before the discovery of AIDS. KS is the most common malignancy in patients who are HIV positive. Prior to the introduction of HAART, KS occurred in nearly 15% of patients with AIDS, but this has decreased dramatically in the age of HAART.

Oral KS in patients not on immunosuppressive therapy is correlated with a lowered CD4 count and is diagnostic for AIDS. Intraorally, KS appears as brown, bluish, purple, or red patches or papules on the hard palate, mucosa, and gingiva. The initial lesions are flat macules or patches on the mucosal surface, but, over time, they become nodular and often

ulcerate and bleed. KS can also manifest on the skin, with lymph node enlargement, and in the salivary glands. Edema commonly occurs in association with extensive cutaneous involvement.

Human herpes-virus 8 (HHV-8) DNA can be found in KS cells and patients with both HIV and HHV-8 infection have a high risk of developing KS. Though oral KS may be the cause of early symptoms, the tumor is usually multifocal, with lesions affecting skin, lymph nodes and viscera. At autopsy most organs are frequently found to be involved.

A biopsy should be performed to definitively diagnose KS. Histologically, KS is characterized by increased vascularity, spindle-shaped cells with little mitotic activity, and hemosiderin deposition. Treatment is accomplished through a variety of methods. Lesions may be injected with sclerosing agents such as vinblastine or sodium tetradecyl sulfate. Advanced cases may require treatment with radiation and/or chemotherapeutic agents such as doxorubicin. The course of the disease can be aggressive, and death due to lung involvement may occur.

12. 1. 4 Herpes Simplex

Herpes simplex virus (HSV) is a double-stranded DNA virus that has 2 subtypes: HSV-1 and HSV-2. Stress, fever, and sunlight may precipitate reactivation of HSV, which usually lies dormant in nearby ganglia. After this stimulus, or decreased immune surveillance, the virus travels down peripheral nerves to produce lesions. The frequency and the severity of these recurrences vary, but the lesions most commonly occur on the vermilion of the lips and are sometimes preceded by a burning or tingling sensation. Numerous small (<1 mm) vesicles appear, which sometimes coalesce into larger vesicles. These then rupture and leave behind painful, weeping ulcerations. These ulcerations are highly infectious until they eventually crust over, which usually takes approximately 3 – 5 days. The normal duration of lesions is 7 – 10 days in immunocompetent individuals.

Immunodeficiency, as seen with HIV disease, permits reactivation of latent herpes infections. Until disproved, all perineal and orolabial ulcerations should be evaluated for HSV in patients who are infected with HIV. Compared with individuals who are immunocompetent, HSV infection in a patient who is HIV positive is more aggressive, prolonged, and diffuse.

Intraoral lesions occur most commonly on the keratinized mucosa, such as the dorsal aspect of the tongue, gingiva, and hard palate. Here, they form single or multiple coalescing vesicles with irregular margins that rupture into ulcerations. Although the keratinized mucosa is usually infected, HSV lesions can manifest on nonkeratinized surfaces in immunocompromised hosts. These include the labial mucosa, ventral tongue, floor of the mouth, buccal mucosa, and the soft palate. Herpetic lesions may extend to other areas, including the tonsillar pillars and the esophagus.

Diagnosis is made by physical examination and a history of prodrome at the site of the vesicles. A Tzanck smear demonstrating multinucleate giant cells is suggestive, but culture and antibody stain results are diagnostic. Tissue biopsy can also be used to obtain a definitive diagnosis. Thymidine kinase inhibitors are the most commonly used antivirals to treat HSV infections. These include acyclovir, valacyclovir, and famciclovir. However, acyclovir-resistant strains are more common among HIV-infected individuals. In these instances, the infections are treated aggressively with intravenous foscarnet.

12. 1. 5   Cytomegalovirus

Cytomegalovirus (CMV) is a double-stranded DNA virus that is fairly common in the general population, with approximately 60% of people being seropositive but asymptomatic. Symptomatic disease does not usually occur unless the patient has undergone organ or bone marrow transplantation, has HIV disease, or is immunocompromised in some other way. CMV retinitis occurs in 30% of patients with AIDS, causing blindness. CMV pneumonia occurs in 5% of patients with AIDS. Pneumonia and adrenalitis due to CMV may be a leading cause of death in patients with AIDS. CMV may also be a cause of subacute encephalitis, resulting in headaches and personality changes in patients with AIDS.

In patients who are immunocompromised, the infection rarely manifests intraorally. However, when it does, CMV produces deep, penetrating oral ulcerations on the lips, tongue, pharynx, or any mucosal site. The aphthouslike ulcerations have a punched-out look with rolled, erythematous borders. Diagnosis is definitive upon detection of the characteristic "owl's eye" appearance of cellular inclusions during the histologic examination. CMV is treated with intravenous agents such as ganciclovir

or cidofovir.

12. 1. 6   Human Papillomavirus

As with the human herpesviruses, human papilloma virus (HPV) infections are more common in individuals with HIV disease. The papillomas or condylomas appear on the gingiva and sometimes the lips and labial mucosa; they are soft pink masses with a characteristic papillary surface texture. These can be treated by excision, laser ablation, or chemical means (e. g. 5-fluorouracil, imiquimod). One study showed that a combination regimen of intralesional and subcutaneous injections of interferon alfa produced resolution of lesions.

Also of interest is that although the incidence of lesions is declining in the age of HAART, most studies agree that the incidence of HPV infection is actually increasing. The reason for this phenomenon is unclear.

12. 1. 7   Aphthouslike Ulcerations

Aphthous ulcerations are ulcerations of the oral cavity that typically cannot be classified as due to any other infectious agent. In immunocompetent individuals, these ulcerations (termed canker sores in the vernacular) usually affect only the nonkeratinized surfaces of the oral cavity. However, in immunocompromised hosts, these ulcerations can appear anywhere. Although 3 forms of recurrent aphthous ulcerations are recognized (i. e. minor, major, herpetiform), the major form is more common in persons with HIV disease. The appearance of these lesions in an HIV-infected patient is a reliable indicator of severe immunodeficiency and disease progression.

Aphthous lesions manifest as yellowish-gray areas of ulceration ranging in size from a few millimeters to larger than a centimeter. The ulcerations are surrounded with a halo of erythema and are usually very painful. Major aphthae are larger than 1 cm in diameter and heal in 14 – 21 days. Major aphthae differ from the other forms of the condition in that they can heal with scarring.

Aphthouslike ulcerations can be treated with a wide array of immune-modulating agents that can be delivered via topical, intralesional, or systemic means. Practitioners should be careful with topical immunosuppressants in this patient population because of the risk of candidal overgrowth that can accompany these agents. Patients who cannot tolerate the adverse effects or additional immunocompromise from the immunosuppressive agents can sometimes be treated with thalidomide.

Because so many conditions in HIV-affected individuals can manifest with ulceration of the oral cavity and because the presentations are often atypical, biopsy is indicated for definitive diagnosis of all HIV-related ulcerations.

12. 2 Gastrointestinal Diseases

The oral cavity is the portal of entry to the GI tract. Lined by stratified squamous epithelium, the tissues of the mouth are often involved when individuals have conditions affecting the GI system. These may be immune-mediated or chemically mediated processes.

12. 2. 1 Crohn Disease

Crohn disease is an idiopathic disorder that can involve the entire GI tract with transmural inflammation, noncaseating granulomas, and fissures. This disease is most common in Western countries and is slightly more prevalent among white males. The peak incidence is in the second and third decades of life, with a second peak occurring in the sixth and seventh decades. Symptoms of Crohn disease include intermittent attacks of diarrhea, constipation, abdominal pain, and fever. Patients may develop malabsorption and subsequent malnutrition. Fissures or fistulas may occur in persons with chronic disease.

Intraoral involvement in Crohn disease occurs in 8%- 9% of patients and may precede intestinal involvement. With oral involvement, the likelihood of extraintestinal manifestations is greater. Extraintestinal features are also common in persons with Crohn disease, and these may manifest systemically as arthritis, clubbing of the fingers, sacroiliitis, and erythema nodosum.

Orofacial symptoms of Crohn disease include ① diffuse labial, gingival, or mucosal swelling; ② cobblestoning of the buccal mucosa and gingiva; ③ aphthous ulcers; ④ mucosal tags; and ⑤ angular cheilitis. Noncaseating granulomas are characteristic of orofacial Crohn disease. Oral granulomas may occur without characteristic alimentary involvement (orofacial granulomatoses). However, the term orofacial granulomatoses encompasses a variety of other disorders, including sarcoidosis, Melkersson-Rosenthal syndrome, and, rarely, tuberculosis. Whether patients with orofacial granulomatoses will subsequently develop intestinal manifestations of Crohn disease is uncertain, but histologic similarities between the oral lesions and the intestinal lesions are obvious. Labial swelling is most often a cosmetic complaint, but it can be a painful manifestation of the disease. Gingival and mucosal involvement may cause difficulty while eating. The pattern of swelling, inflammation, ulcers, and fissures is similar to that of the lesions occurring in the intestinal tract. Acute and chronic inflammation, with lymphocytic and giant cell perivascular infiltrates, and lymphoid follicles are the most common histologic findings in oral and GI Crohn disease. Noncaseating granulomas are present in biopsy samples in a number of cases. Increased dental caries and nutritional deficiencies may be related to decreased saliva production and malabsorption in the intestinal tract.

Oral findings as described above warrant a full systemic evaluation for intestinal Crohn disease, including referral for colonoscopy and biopsy with histopathologic correlation. Oral involvement may precede systemic manifestations and symptoms. Negative findings on GI evaluations should be repeated in patients with oral symptoms. The severity of oral lesions may coincide with the severity of the systemic disease, and it may be used as a marker for intestinal impairment.

12. 2. 2 Ulcerative Colitis

Ulcerative colitis is an inflammatory condition with some similarities to Crohn disease. However, it is restricted to the colon and is limited to the mucosa and submucosa, sparing the muscularis. Lesions in the colon consist of areas of hemorrhage and ulcerations along with abscesses. Similar lesions may manifest in the oral cavity as aphthous ulcerations or superficial hemorrhagic ulcers. Ulcerative colitis is characterized by periods of exacerbation and remission, and, generally, oral lesions coincide with exacerbations of the colonic disease. Similar ulcerations may arise on the buttocks, abdomen, thighs, and face. Aphthous ulcers or angular stomatitis occurs in as many as 5%- 10% of patients.

12. 2. 3 Gastroesophageal Reflux

Gastroesophageal reflux disease (GERD) is a common condition. Regurgitation of gastric contents (pH 1 - 2) reduces the pH of the oral cavity below 5. 5; this acidic pH begins to dissolve enamel. It is most commonly seen on the palatal surfaces of the maxillary dentition. Erosion of the enamel exposes the underlying dentin, which is a softer, more yellow, material. The extent of erosion depends on the frequency and the quantity of exposure along with the duration of disease. Newly exposed dentin is smooth and shiny, while dentin from previous exposures may be stained. Exposed dentin is often sensitive to temperature changes and, secondary to its lower mineral content, develops caries much more quickly.

Erosion differs from dental caries in that it is a hard, dished-out area where enamel has dissolved and the underlying dentin is exposed. On the other hand, caries reveals soft, discolored dentin and results from the bacterial breakdown of sugars into acid, which demineralizes the surface of the teeth. The prevalence of caries is not increased in persons with GERD, possibly because the acidic environment interferes with the formation of the dental biofilm, or the good dental care and control of acid help decrease the prevalence of erosion. However, once the erosion occurs, it is irreversible and can only be treated with surgical restorative procedures. Therefore, early recognition and patient education is the most effective treatment.

12.2.4 Chronic Liver Disease

Chronic liver disease impacts many systems of the body. The coagulation pathway is one such system. The liver synthesizes many of the clotting factors necessary for hemostasis. In addition, vitamin K, a fat-soluble vitamin, requires proper liver function to be adequately absorbed from the intestines. In patients with liver disease, the resultant impaired hemostasis can be manifested in the mouth as petechiae or excessive gingival bleeding with minor trauma. This is especially suggestive if it occurs in the absence of inflammation. Therefore, special care must be taken during any type of surgery, oral or otherwise; severe hemorrhage can ensue as a result of the paucity of clotting factors.

The only manifestation of advanced liver disease visible in the oral mucosa is jaundice, which is the yellow pigmentation that results from the deposition of bilirubin in the submucosa. Jaundice may occur following disorders in bilirubin metabolism, production, or secretion. Hepatocellular damage affects secretion, the rate-limiting step in bilirubin metabolism, allowing conjugated bilirubin to leak out of the cells and into the blood stream. This water-soluble substance is loosely albumin bound, and it is deposited in the mucous membranes throughout the body. When jaundice is due to chronic liver disease, the yellow color reflects a direct relation to liver function. Jaundice manifests at serum levels greater than 2.5 – 3 mg/dL or 2 – 3 times baseline. Because they are thinner, the mucosa on the soft palate and in the sublingual region are often first to reveal a yellow hue. With time, the yellow changes can be visible at any mucosal site.

Because of its high rate of progression to chronic hepatitis (50%) and cirrhosis, hepatitis C is the leading infectious cause of chronic liver disease worldwide. The association between hepatitis C and oral lichen planus is controversial. This association is greater in Europe and Asia than it is in the United States, where no significant correlation has been noted. The link between the two conditions is tenuous and not sufficient to warrant screening for hepatitis C infection in all patients with lichen planus.

12.3 Hematologic Disorders

12.3.1 Anemia

The potential causes for reduction in oxygen-carrying capacity are legion. Fatigue and decreased resistance to infection are common systemic symptoms. The nail beds and oral mucosa exhibit pallor. This pallor is a common and easily recognizable feature of anemia.

Mucosal conditions, such as glossitis, recurrent aphthae, candidal infections, and angular stomatitis may be more common in patients with anemia. Glossitis may be the first sign of folate or vitamin B-12 deficiency. The tongue appears reddened, and the papillae are atrophic, producing a smooth ("bald") appearance. Angular stomatitis is commonly caused by a candidal infection, and it has been linked to iron deficiency. If the anemia persists, resistance to infection may be decreased.

12.3.2 Langerhans Cell Histiocytosis

Langerhans cell histiocytosis has replaced the term histiocytosis X, a condition of unknown etiology and pathogenesis characterized by abnormal proliferation of histiocytes and eosinophils. Langerhans cell histiocytosis may manifest with either localized proliferation or more extensive systemic involvement.

One form, previously referred to as Letterer-Siwe disease, is most common in infants and is characterized by widespread involvement of the viscera, potentially leading to death. Skin lesions are common and include papules, plaques, vesicles, and hemorrhagic nodules, all of which may manifest in a pattern similar to that of seborrheic dermatitis. Oral symptoms include large ulcerations, ecchymoses, gingivitis, periodontitis, and subsequent tooth loss.

A more localized variant, primarily referred to as Hand-Schüller-Christian disease, is a childhood disease that consists of the triad of diabetes insipidus, lytic bone lesions, and proptosis. Oral manifestations include irregular ulcerations of the hard palate, which may be the primary manifestation of the disease. Gingival inflammation and ulcerated nodules, difficulty in chewing, and foul-smelling breath also occur.

The most common form of Langerhans cell histiocytosis is the eosinophilic granuloma type, which develops in young adults. Radiolucent bone lesions can occur anywhere but are most common in flat bones, such as the posterior jaw. Radiologic findings demonstrate rapid progressive alveolar bone loss with dental extrusion, producing the characteristic appearance of "floating teeth." These lesions result in fractures and displaced teeth.

Oral swellings or ulcerations resulting from mandibular or maxillary bone involvement are common. Oral ulcerations may develop on the gingiva, palate, and floor of the mouth, along with a necrotizing gingivitis. Oral lesions may occur without underlying bone destruction. In these rare cases, ulceration of the palate or gingiva may be the primary oral sign.

A biopsy specimen reveals the pale Langerhans cells with bilobed nuclei, which resemble coffee beans. Clusters of eosinophils also may be present. Biopsy is necessary and should be used for diagnosis because the ulcerations are nonspecific.

12. 4 Connective-tissue Disorders

12. 4. 1 Sjögren Syndrome
Sjögren syndrome is the second most common autoimmune disease, affecting as many as 3% of women aged 50 years or older. The sex predilection is profound: approximately 90% of patients are female. Sjögren syndrome is characterized by Sicca syndrome, keratoconjunctivitis Sicca, and xerostomia. A secondary form is associated with rheumatoid arthritis.

Oral changes in Sjögren syndrome include difficulty in swallowing and eating, disturbances in taste and speech, increased dental caries, and a predisposition to infection, all due to a decrease in saliva. These changes are nonspecific for Sjögren syndrome because they may occur in any condition associated with diminished saliva production. Saliva can be thick, ropey, and mucinous, or it may be altogether absent. The mucosal changes typical of xerostomia include dry, red, and wrinkled mucosa. The tongue may exhibit a cobblestonelike appearance due to atrophy of the papillae. Candidiasis is common in persons with Sjögren syndrome. An increased incidence of dental caries is also common of Sjögren syndrome because the amount of saliva is insufficient to rinse away or dilute dietary sugar and the buffering capacity is greatly reduced.

Histologic examination of minor salivary or lacrimal glands reveals the cause for this decrease in saliva and tears. In Sjögren syndrome, lymphocytic infiltrates surround the salivary gland and lacrimal gland ducts. The inflammation and resultant epithelial hyperplasia render the ducts blocked and useless. This leads to atrophy of the acini, fibrosis, and hyalinization of the gland. These changes are irreversible, although certain medications can help to maximize saliva production from the remaining functional glandular tissue. Taken together, these facts reinforce the philosophy that good oral hygiene and frequent dental visits are essential in minimize the deleterious effects of compromised salivary flow.

12. 4. 2 Reiter Syndrome
Reiter syndrome is a common cause of inflammatory oligoarthropathy in young male patients. The arthritis is accompanied by conjunctivitis and urethritis. An association with HLA-B27 and chlamydia urethritis or Shigella dysentery has been demonstrated. A common symptom of Reiter syndrome is superficial ulceration of the buccal mucosa, which is usually transient and asymptomatic.

12. 4. 3 Kawasaki Disease
Kawasaki disease, or mucocutaneous lymph node syndrome, is a vasculitis that affects medium and large arteries with a corresponding cutaneous lymph node syndrome. Kawasaki disease has replaced rheumatic fever as the primary cause of childhood heart disease in the United States. Children younger than

5 years are most commonly affected. Patients present acutely with edema, erythema of the hands and feet, fever, oral erythema, and rash. The associated temperature must exceed 38.5℃ (101.3℉) for 5 days to meet diagnostic criteria.

For diagnosis, 4 of the 5 following criteria must also be met: ① peripheral extremity edema, erythema, or desquamation; ② polymorphous exanthem; ③ bilateral conjunctival injection; ④ erythema and strawberry tongue in the oral cavity; and ⑤ acute cervical adenopathy. Cardiac sequelae to the vasculitis may result in aneurysm and myocardial infarction. Myocarditis commonly occurs within a week after the fever. Within 2 - 3 weeks, the previously edematous palms and soles peel and slough.

Oral findings include swelling of papillae on the surface of the tongue (strawberry tongue) and intense erythema of the mucosal surfaces. The labia are cracked, cherry red, swollen, and hemorrhagic. The last of these may be due to the long-standing high-grade fevers.

■ Summary

Many systemic disorders have oral manifestations. The oral component may precede the systemic presentation of a particular disease. Early diagnosis and management can often diminish the morbidity associated with a systemic disease. Careful examination of the oral cavity is a necessary component of the diagnostic work-up for any patient.

■ Questions

1. What is the oral manifestation of HIV disease?

2. How many kinds of systemic diseases could lead to the oral ulceration?

3. What conditions of gastrointestinal system would affect the tissues of mouth?

4. What oral changes are there in Sjögren syndrome?

5. What oral effects and clinical features are there in Hematologic Disorders?

(**Jingping Bai** 柏景坪)

References

[1] Slavkin HC, Baum BJ. Relationship of dental and oral pathology to systemic illness. JAMA, 2000, 284:1215-1217.

[2] Nokta M. Oral manifestations associated with HIV infection. Curr HIV/AIDS Rep, 2008, 5(1):5-12.

[3] Reznik DA. Oral manifestations of HIV disease. Top HIV Med, 2005, 13(5):143-148.

[4] Feller L, Lemmer J, Wood NH, et al. HIV-associated oral Kaposi sarcoma and HHV-8: a review. J Int Acad Periodontol, 2007, 9(4):129-136.

[5] Fiasse R, Denis MA, Dewit O. Chronic inflammatory bowel disease: Crohn's disease and ulcerative colitis. J Pharm Belg, 2010, 1:1-9.

[6] Gorsky M, Eptsein JB. A case series of acquired immunodeficiency syndrome patients with initial neoplastic diagnoses of intraoral Kaposi's sarcoma. Med Oral Pathol Oral Radiol Endod, 2000, 90:612-617.

[7] Biel K, Bohm M, Luger TA, et al. Long-standing aphthae-a clue to the diagnosis of coeliac disease. Dermatology, 2000, 200:340.

[8] Alfaro EV, Aps JK, Martens LC. Oral implications in children with gastroesophageal reflux disease. Curr Opin Pediatr, 2008, 20(5):576-583.

[9] Blumin JH, Merati AL, Toohill RJ. Duodenogastroesophageal reflux and its effect on extraesophageal tissues: a review. Ear Nose Throat J, 2008, 87(4):234-237.

[10] Pace F, Pallotta S, Tonini M, et al. Systematic review: gastro-oesophageal reflux disease and dental lesions. Aliment Pharmacol Ther, 2008, 27(12):1179-1186.

[11] Vassilopoulos D, Manolakopoulos S. Rheumatic manifestations of hepatitis. Curr Opin Rheumatol, 2010, 22(1):91-96.

[12] Madrigal-Martínez-Pereda C, Guerrero-Rodríguez V, Guisado-Moya B, et al. Langerhans cell histiocytosis: literature review and descriptive analysis of oral manifestations. Med Oral Patol Oral Cir Bucal, 2009, 14(5): E222-228.

[13] Hernández-Juyol M, Boj-Quesada JR, Gallego Melcon S. Oral manifestations of Langerhans cell histiocytosis. Case study of a two-year-old boy. Med Oral, 2003, 8(1):19-25.

[14] Margaix-Muñoz M, Bagán JV, Poveda R, et al. Sjögren's syndrome of the oral cavity. Review and update. Med Oral Patol Oral Cir Bucal, 2009, 14(7):E325-330.

[15] Mathews SA, Kurien BT, Scofield RH. Oral manifestations of Sjögren's syndrome. J Dent Res, 2008, 87(4): 308-318.

[16] Cummings NA. The oral-mucosal manifestations of rheumatic diseases. Rheumatology, 1973, 4(0):60-97.

[17] Kim DS. Kawasaki disease. Yonsei Med J, 2006, 47(6): 759-772.

[18] Mendoza N, Diamantis M, Arora A, et al. Mucocutaneous manifestations of Epstein-Barr virus infection. Am J Clin Dermatol, 2008, 9(5):295-305.

[19] Callen JP. Oral manifestations of collagen vascular disease. Semin Cutan Med Surg, 1997, 16:323-327.

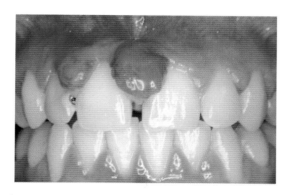

Color Figure 3-1   Pregnancy-associated
pyogenic granuloma

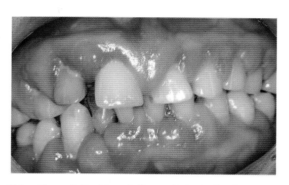

Color Figure 3-2   Drug-influenced gingival enlargement

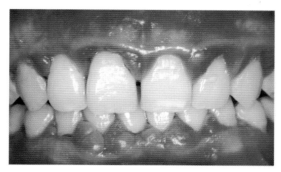

Color Figure 3-3   Highly visible changes in gingiva

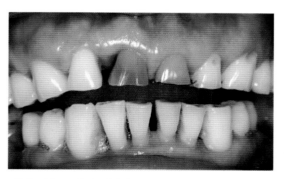

Color Figure 3-4   Minimal visible changes in gingiva

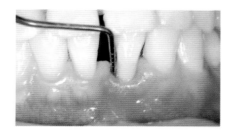
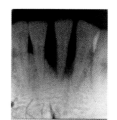
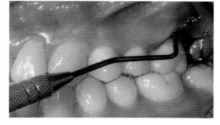
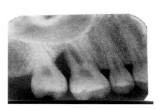

Color Figure 3-5   Localized aggressive periodontitis

2

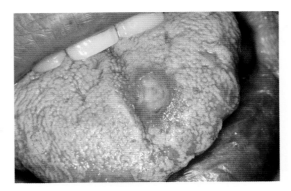

Color Figure 4-1   Minor aphthous ulcers on the tongue

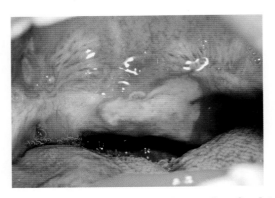

Color Figure 4-2   Major aphthous ulcers on the soft palate

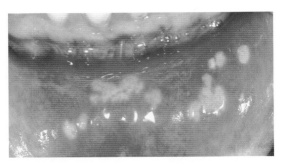

Color Figure 4-3   Herpetiform ulcers on the labial mucosa

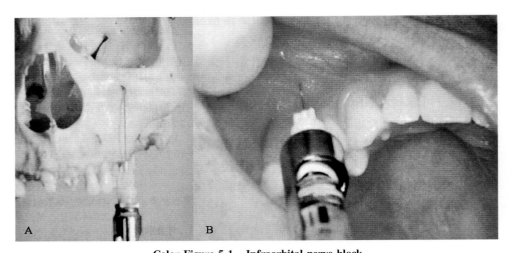

Color Figure 5-1   Infraorbital nerve block
A. Proper position of the needle and syringe. B. Insertion of the needle at the crest of the mucobuccal fold
adjacent to the axillary first bicuspid

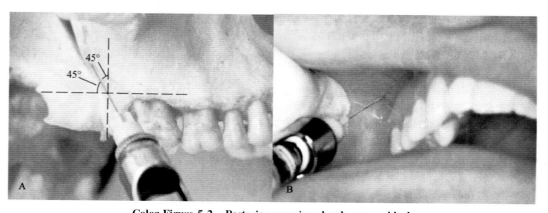

Color Figure 5-2   Posterior-superior alveolar nerve block
A. Proper position of the needle and syringe. B. Insertion of the needle at height of mucobuccal fold
at the maxillary second-third molar region

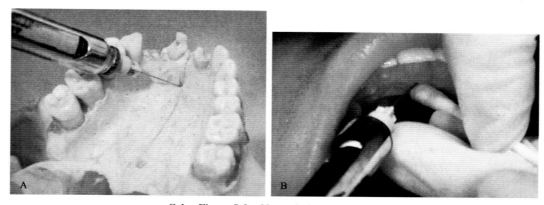

Color Figure 5-3   Nasopalatine nerve block
A. Proper position of the needle and syringe. B. Insertion of the needle from the lateral
aspect of the incisive papillae toward the incisive canal

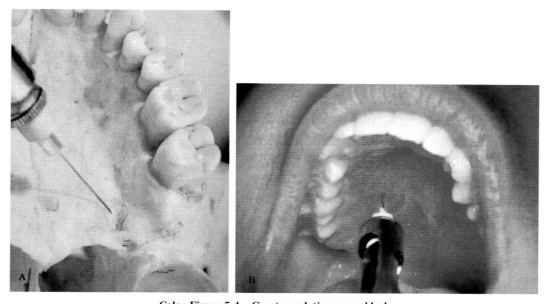

Color Figure 5-4   Greater palatine nerve block
A. Proper position of the needle and syringe. B. Needle penetrating the
lateral palatal vault in proximity to the maxillary third molar

4

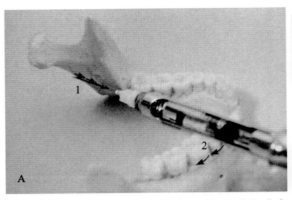
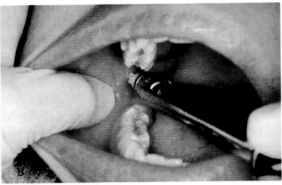

Color Figure 5-5   Inferior alveolar nerve block
A. Proper position of the needle and syringe. B. Insertion of the needle
lateral to the pterygomandibular raphe approximately 1 cm above the occlusal plane

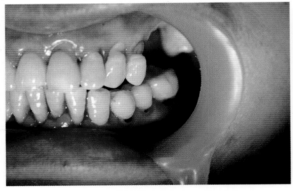

**Color Figure 11-1   Root surfaces exposed and root
surface caries**

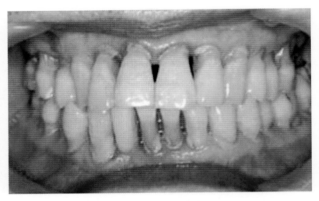

Color Figure 11-2   Severity of periodontal diseases of elderly

N3-04-05